Wellness Recovery Action Plan

&

Peer Support

Wellness Recovery Action Plan

&

Peer Support

Personal, Group and Program Development

by Mary Ellen Copeland & Shery Mead

Peach
Press
Dummerston, Vermont

Publishers Note

This publication is designed to provide accurate and authoritative information in regard to the subject matter covered. It is sold with the understanding that the publisher is not engaged in rendering psychological, financial, legal, or other professional services. If expert assistance or counseling is needed, the services of a competent professional should be sought.

❦ Dedications ❦

This book is dedicated to the memory of my nephew, Paul Copeland, who ended his life in 1993. I am convinced that, if services and options like the ones described in this book had been available to Paul, he would be alive today.
—*Mary Ellen Copeland*

It is also dedicated to Ashley, Casey and Russell for making me "walk the talk" every single day.
—*Shery Mead*

And it is dedicated to the memory of David Hilton, who challenged us all to think "outside the box."

Contents

🦪

Appendices

Foreword

Let us imagine for a moment that we have given ourselves permission to take a good chunk of the time and energy we spend in systems, and turn it toward building healing communities and wellness plans. What would happen if we surrounded ourselves with people who exuded hope for our future and valued being mutually responsible to one another? What if everyone was encouraged to discover the expertise they had to offer and was given the opportunity to share their knowledge and skills? What would be the result of placing our faith in the common wisdom of our community and focusing attention on new ways of thinking about our experiences?

Pairing the philosophies and tools of a trauma-informed approach to peer support with Wellness Recovery Action Planning (WRAP), this manual provides a guide to exploring the possibilities of personal well-being through community. It is a compelling package of theory and practice. The curriculum provides readers with a new way of teaching and exploring WRAP within the safety of mutually supportive peer relationships. Audiences of all kinds will find the exercises and concrete skills transferable to their situations. Peer support groups, self-help networks, individuals, families, and all sorts of practitioners will benefit from the contents of this manual.

Over the years I have studied many mental health initiatives and the cumulative evidence indicates that peer support and WRAP offer a powerful health-oriented alternative to traditional practices. WRAP has had a great deal of positive influence in the lives of people who are committed to working on their well-being. This is evidenced by its tremendous use and the volumes of success stories that people have to offer. Peer support communities are providing a caring haven for many. Studies of these programs indicate that the helping relationships and healing strategies offered by peers are qualitatively different than those encountered in other professional interactions.

However, we live in an era where the credibility of a program or practice is grounded in the ability to demonstrate empirical outcomes, and as such, the time has come for peer programs to step up to the plate. Making the impacts of peer support and WRAP empirical will require a discovery process across many different kinds of peer communities. Investigations need to be conducted in a manner that reflects the theory, practices and values of peer support and WRAP.

Fitting with the tradition of peer support and WRAP, future studies will have to propose different kinds of questions and challenge assumptions - assumptions about what is important to know, how to go about the knowing, and how to best represent what has been learned. Only in this way will we realize and help others to appreciate what it is that makes WRAP and peer support a distinct form of help.

The writings of Mary Ellen Copeland and Shery Mead show us a way of redefining the problem and provide us with practical strategies for enhancing our well-being. 'It's NOT all in your head…it's all around you!' is the basic premise of their message. Let us celebrate the hope and the possibilities that these authors have to share. And let us find ways in which we can help others to understand what we are coming to know.

Cheryl MacNeil, Ph.D.

Research and Evaluation Consultant

macred@capital.net

From the Authors

Mary Ellen Copeland

This book is a next step. It goes beyond all that I have learned in my studies of how people cope with difficulties on a day-to-day basis. It goes beyond WRAP. It goes beyond Peer Support. It is about developing and using WRAP together with Peer Support methodologies that are "trauma informed" to challenge our old ways of thinking and broaden our perspectives. Combining these two strategies helps us not only to recover, but also to change our perceptions of ourselves from "sick mental patient" to healthy people; to learn how to build sustaining relationships with others and to develop healthy patterns of growth and change that will support us through our lives.

As many of you already know, recovery from what have been known as psychiatric symptoms, (what I now prefer to refer to as difficult times), is my passion. I care deeply about recovery because difficult times and a system that didn't understand stole eight years of my mother's life and many years of my life. My mother found her way back (with little help) and so did I. Many others are now finding their way out and going on to lead happy lives. But there are still millions of people around the world who are living out their lives believing they can never recover and that what has happened is their fault. Their lives are frustrating and often unfulfilled. Many of them live in institutions, supported housing or long-term care homes. Some are in jails or prisons. Many live on the streets and in deep poverty. Far too often they are treated badly by family members and people who are supposed to be providing them with care and safety.

Not so many years ago, my life fell apart. I felt deeply sad almost all of the time. I thought I had no value—that I was hopeless and worthless. My anxiety was often so intense that I felt immobilized. Flashbacks haunted both my waking and sleeping hours. I responded to others and the circumstances of my life being out of control with anger and fear. I isolated myself. I often hurt myself, sabotaged myself and repeatedly tried to end my life. It felt like my life was over and I was descending into the pits of hell. My only relief was brief periods of elation, but sometimes I got "too elated" and did things I wish I had never done, spent money I didn't have and embarrassed myself in my community.

Care providers told me I was mentally ill, like my mother. They said that I had to take medication for the rest of my life in order to get better. And for a long time I bought that view, as unhelpful as it was. They never asked me what had happened to me in my life. They never asked me what my life was like. There was no mention of the sexual abuse I experienced as a child and the troubled relationships that plagued my adulthood. And, there was no mention of the on-going trauma I was experiencing in the mental health system.

Slowly I dug myself out of the hole and began working on my recovery. There have been times when my progress seemed interminably slow—almost stagnant. And then I would learn something new and feel like I was moving ahead at the speed of light. Those moments when the change has seemed so accelerated were when I realized things like:

- There is lots of hope—people like me can and do recover and move on with their lives.
- I am a worthwhile, special, unique person who deserves all the best that life has to offer.
- I have more strengths and resources than I ever imagined.
- I can take back control of my life and do things to help myself.
- There are numerous simple and safe things I can do to help myself.
- I can learn from others who have had similar experiences.
- The bad things that have happened in my life have affected all of my life,
- causing me to feel badly about myself and affecting the ways I relate and respond to others.
- I can overcome the effects of trauma and continue to work toward wellness.
- I can change trauma-based responses to responses based on what is really happening in my world now.
- I can develop and use a WRAP to guide and sustain my wellness.
- I can have rich and fulfilling relationships.

I hope that as you read this book, and make changes in your life and/or program based on what you have learned, you will have many times when you feel like you too are progressing at the speed of light.

Shery Mead

The concept of Peer Support that you will be reading about in this book is very personal for me. In fact, without it in my life, I would never have moved beyond my own "mental patient" role. Let me explain. For most of my life, I lived "on the edge." I thought about things differently than other people, acted in ways that landed me in psychiatric settings, and felt pretty alone, isolated, with a strong sense of "other-than-ness," like somehow I was defective, bad, and probably not good for others.

At 17, after some particularly difficult experiences, I ended up in a locked psychiatric unit where I was told that I had something called "schizophrenia," (a popular diagnosis in the late 60's). This was basically the same message that was given to my fellow patients, so I began to adopt the cultural "truths" of this environment. I listened to the doctor when he said that I needed to take Thorazine, and I didn't resist when he suggested shock treatments. Luckily for me, I didn't agree to move into the recommended "halfway house," but I certainly did hold on to the "mental patient" identity that they had created for me.

For years, I carried around the notion that something was terribly wrong with me. It deeply affected what I thought I was capable of, and it led me into some very abusive relationships. I honestly thought that I deserved bad treatment, and was always surprised when people were kind and caring. It wasn't until I had children of my own that I began to see the toll all of these messages had taken. Further, I recognized that "my messages" stood to contribute to my own children's lives if I didn't change.

I was very lucky to find a practitioner who saw things from a different perspective. She was never judgmental, nor did she ever see me as "sick." In fact, even when I was at my worst and tried to convince her I was "sick," she wouldn't buy it. This was not true in the rest of the field. When, as an adult, I ended up back in psychiatric hospitals, I was told once again that I had a serious mental illness and that I might as well let go of the things I had begun to aspire to. For years, this culture of illness won out, in spite of my practitioner's best efforts.

It wasn't until I began advocating for women in a domestic violence program that I finally began to realize the devastating impact of this illness culture, and of psychiatric labeling, on so many other women. Over and over, women who were being abused and who sought mental health treatment were told that they had a psychiatric illness. They were told that they should give up custody of their children because of their illnesses, told they needed medication and therapy, and then told that they couldn't talk about their abuse because it was not relevant to their mental illness. I watched women, once again, having their reality defined for them.

And so I fought. I argued with psychiatrists, mental health practitioners, and, finally, the state department of mental health, where I found out about some potential funding for Peer Support. Although at the time I wasn't sure what Peer Support meant, I absolutely believed that we could create something to help people understand the profound effects of abuse, and what that meant to how they saw themselves. I was sure that we could finally help people start to build supportive relationships and communities where they could talk about whatever they needed to talk about without being judged, further labeled, or disbelieved.

It didn't take long, however, before we realized that it would take a lot of practice not to continue to do what had been done to us. After all, it's easy to fall back into using power and control when you're uncomfortable, and it's not always easy to support people in finding their personal strengths while learning together. We decided that we would need to develop our own training rather than count on any of the traditional "helping" models, and so we talked about what it meant to share responsibility, to maintain mutuality, and to create a "culture of health and ability."

It was at this time that the language of recovery was just beginning to be introduced and those of us at the peer center wanted to make sure that we were in on the ground floor of defining it! We also wanted to make sure that the system became more aware of the impact of trauma and abuse on people's mental health. Not only familial abuse, but also the traumatizing effects of "treatments" like seclusion and restraints. In fact, we became more and more clear that much of the "mental patient" role was being perpetuated by the mental health system and particularly by psychiatric hospitals.

We decided to start a peer run hospital alternative. We began to learn more about what it really meant to "hear" the story of the other person, while at the same time working diligently to share responsibility and maintain mutuality even in very difficult situations.

It's clear to me, after teaching Peer Support widely around the country, that we can't stop now. Too often, we are falling into old roles and relationships with one another. We are adopting clinical-type interactions with each other (even if we don't use "their" language), and we are hurting each other with judgment, gossip, and abuses of power. In other words, without maintaining a constant awareness, we are doing what many organizations do.

I am hopeful that this book can contribute to the practice and maintenance of true Peer Support. I hope that we can continue to learn what that means and evolve it without becoming tied to any particular way of doing things. AND I hope we can be proud of what we've accomplished and what Peer Support has meant to our lives, our relationships, and to our communities. I know it's totally changed my life and I hope the lives of my children and potential grandchildren! As I've been known to say: "So long as we challenge how we've come to 'know what we know,' we can change the world."

> *Note:* Throughout this book we will be referring to "staff" roles. Staff, in this case, refers to people (whether paid or unpaid) who have agreed to be accountable for certain responsibilities in their peer program or group (director, bookkeeper, warmline worker, group facilitator, etc.) Other than making sure these responsibilities are carried out, we understand the role of staff as maintaining and modeling Peer Support values (See WRAP and Peer Support Values in Chapter 2) in all aspects of the program. We also recognize that staff language, in and of itself, sets up a hierarchical relationship and so we must constantly reflect on how those dynamics play out in Peer Support. Whether your program has paid staff, volunteer staff, or is a collaborative effort, our goal is to make sure that we are truly doing what we say we're doing.

Chapter 1

Why WRAP & Peer Support?

The Wellness Recovery Action Plan is recognized as an exemplary practice that has been widely accepted and used since its development in 1997 by a group of people who used mental health services. Until recently, WRAP plans were just tools for individuals to use to identify the resources they could use to stay well, to work through difficult times and to assist them in their recovery and personal growth. As a recovery aid, WRAP is quite straightforward and has been tremendously successful.

Peer Support has not been quite as concrete. Although there are many kinds of peer programs and services, we've yet to establish a way of thinking that makes Peer Support uniform. Peer Support may mean one thing to one person and something else to another. We can agree that Peer Support offers many people another way to think about mental health and help, and an opportunity to build mutually responsible, mutually supportive relationships. Peer Support gives people an opportunity to explore who they've become, how their self-perception may be limiting them, and help them to see themselves, and all that's possible, in a new way.

Another way of looking at the relationship between Peer Support and Wellness Recovery Action Planning is that Peer Support allows us to create relationships with others in new and different ways that promote growth, recovery and wellness. WRAP gives us a way to lead our lives in new and different ways that promote growth, recovery and wellness. The skills and strategies that we discover in Peer Support can become part of our WRAP and the skills and strategies we discover as we use WRAP can assist us in Peer Support.

The combination of WRAP and Peer Support can be incredibly powerful in helping us grow, learn from each other, and challenge each other beyond what we thought we were capable of. Using Peer Support theory with WRAP, we can discover false beliefs about ourselves, and then help each other develop plans and take action to make our lives be the way we want them to be. Both WRAP and Peer Support make space for individual and group growth and healing.

Some of the other reasons that WRAP and Peer Support work well together include:

- They share similar values, ethics, goals and objectives, including self-determination and personal empowerment.
- Peer Support centers and other places where peers gather are ideal places for learning more about both WRAP and Peer Support.
- Peers support each other in developing Wellness Recovery Action Plans in ways that contribute to mutual knowledge and growth, supporting and challenging each other as we work on our recovery.

8| WRAP & Peer Support

- WRAP and Peer Support together can help us discover new ways for handling difficult times that support growth and recovery.
- WRAP and Peer Support challenge old ways of thinking and create new ways of thinking.
- Both strategies are cost effective—There are few costs related to implementation, and research findings are beginning to show that those of us who use these strategies have less need for costly, intensive and invasive treatments.
- They increase the use of natural supports and decrease dependence on system supports.
- They help people develop a realistic understanding of the devastating effects of trauma and abuse.

You may be able to think of other reasons why Peer Support and WRAP work well when used together. If so, you can list them here:

_____

_____

_____

_____

The first section of this book is about **Peer Support.** In it we will explore:

1) New ways of thinking about Peer Support
2) Skills for practicing Peer Support,
3) Methods that help us become more sensitive to the effects of trauma and abuse on our lives, programs, and groups
4) Issues of power and conflict
5) An evaluation method that will help maintain the integrity of our programs and offer evidence of our success.

The section on **Wellness Recovery Action Planning** will describe:

1) What Wellness Recovery Action Planning is
2) Why we "do" WRAP and Peer Support together
3) The values and ethics that are common to both WRAP and Peer Support
4) General guidelines for developing and using WRAP, including specific instructions
5) Follow-up groups
6) Evaluation

This manual includes questions and activities that will stimulate thinking and discussions with others about who we are, how we relate to others, what it means to be a peer, what it means to help, and what we might need to learn to put Peer Support and WRAP values into action. It is our hope that by the end of the book, you will understand how these concepts fit together and how they fit into your life, relationships, and in your program. Read it slowly, have fun, and then put it into action!

Important Considerations

Peer Support and WRAP are for anyone who wants to use them. All too often, people have said that these programs are only for "high functioning" people (whoever *they* are!) or for people who have been given a particular diagnosis. We find this kind of thinking and language to be disrespectful, inaccurate, and judgmental. People have started their journeys to recovery when they were unable to speak or could only mutter, when they were hearing voices constantly, when they were having difficulty sitting still for even a moment, when they had not moved at all for a very long time, and when they have been diagnosed with any psychiatric disorder. And they've begun where they were, perhaps making only very small changes at first. It continues to be exhilarating to be closely connected to people who have taken their first steps and gradually, over time, taken back control of their lives and moved on to work toward meeting their personal goals and dreams.

It is our hope that, as more and more of us are involved in Peer Support and WRAP programs, we will see:

1) More of us building communities of peers and able to meet life and vocational goals, significant life enhancement, and gains in self-esteem and self-confidence as we become valued members of the community

2) A shift of focus in mental health care from symptom control to prevention, personal growth, and recovery

3) A much broader understanding of mental illness and recovery, as well as decreases in discrimination and stigma

4) A significant reduction in the need for mental health and emergency services that are costly, not helpful or healthy, and are often traumatizing.

Chapter 2

What is Peer Support?

A bout ten years ago I (Shery) became the director of a brand new Peer Support program in New Hampshire. Though I had some ideas about what it might look like, I never dreamed that it would involve such a complex process. I soon discovered that if we were going to make this something really different, it would take a tremendous amount of attention and exploration. For me this meant in-depth reading about the peer and mental health recovery movement as well as literature in the fields of feminism, sociology, anthropology and even philosophy. These perspectives helped me avoid falling into the typical mental health traps and assumptions like "people never get well" and "they can't control themselves". It also meant figuring out what values really defined Peer Support and how to integrate them into every aspect of the program. This was not an easy process. It took persistence, patience, and humility. Little by little we were really creating something unique.

Peer Support: A Working Definition

Many of us who have spent a long time in the mental health system have learned roles that support our "patienthood." For instance, after we've been diagnosed and begun to use services, we have often felt like second-class citizens, and began to think about all aspects of our lives through the eyes of "mental patients." We have become, in our own minds, and the mind of others, just a diagnosis, rather than powerful women/men, artists, writers, educators and parents. We've felt ostracized from the community and of little value. This kind of identity has led us to think that the rest of the community can't understand us. This creates an "us/them" split, where we don't feel part of the community and others don't consider us members of the community. Recovery in Peer Support comes through seeing ourselves as human beings, the same as any one else, rather than as mental patients. We begin to do this by practicing relationships in Peer Support in a different way.

Instead of taking care of each other and thinking of each other as "sick," in Peer Support we build a sense of family and community that is mutually responsible and focused on recovery and social action.

Peer Support is not like clinical support, and it is more that just being friends. In Peer Support we understand each other because we've "been there," shared similar experiences and can model for each other a willingness to learn and grow. We come together with the intention of changing unhelpful patterns, getting out of "stuck" places, and building relationships that are respectful, mutually responsible, and, potentially, mutually transforming. At first we may come to a program or center because it feels safe and accepting, but we find that just by sharing our experiences and building trust we are helping each other move beyond our perceived limitations, old patterns, and ways of thinking about our mental health and the mental health of others. This allows us to try out new behaviors with one another and move beyond the "illness culture" where we are defined as "sick" and disabled into a culture of health and ability.

In starting the peer center we quickly realized how challenging it would be to embrace this definition due to the tremendous influence traditional services and assumptions had on us. Even with our best efforts it was not uncommon to see us doing to each other what had been done to us in the past. For example I heard people trying to "help" each other by suggesting more medication, by getting together behind closed doors and "figuring out" what to do with a "difficult" member, or by being condescending and controlling towards one another. We knew it would be important to determine what Peer Support was and what it was not.

How is Peer Support different from other services?

Peer Support is:	*Peer Support is not:*
Being open to new ways of thinking about our experience	An expert telling you what your experience means
Re-defining help and helping	Telling someone what to do
A way of thinking about relationships and power that is mutual	Superficial power-down relationships
Considering the effects of trauma and abuse on people's self-concept and relationships	Telling you you're sick and socially unacceptable
Mutually supportive and mutually responsible	One way relationships where one person takes responsibility for the other
Teaching and learning from each other	Being told or learning about diagnosis and treatment
An opportunity to challenge the status quo	Protecting people from taking risks that are "too stressful.
About recovery and transformation	About stability and maintenance.

What has Peer Support meant to you in your life?

_____

_____

_____

_____

How has it been different than traditional mental health services?

_____

_____

_____

_____

Starting Out

When we first opened the center, it became clear that people who'd been in the mental health system for a long time had formed certain roles and beliefs. Through the years they had been told what they "had," how it should be treated, and to expect lifelong mental health treatment. For example, one man told me that he had been a chronic schizophrenic since the age of fourteen. He proceeded to tell me about the insulin shock treatments, the various state hospitals, and then he told me that he would never get better. He believed that in order to stay "functional" he'd have to depend on clinical help and psychotropic medications for the rest of his life. He had no language for talking about recovery and virtually no hope for a different kind of life. Basically, he had just learned to cope, and led a pretty uninteresting existence: case management appointments, weekly meeting with his payee, and monthly visits with the psychiatrist. Over the years he had gotten used to telling his illness story again and again as if that's all there were to his existence. In other words, he had taken on the role of the "mental patient."

In order to unlearn the mental patient role we must first take a step back and think about how we have adopted it. How did we learn that we were "mentally ill?" When did we start to see ourselves as different from other people?

I've often told the following story of my own "learning to be a mental patient:"

When I was four, I found it much easier to communicate with chipmunks. I talked with them and they spoke with me. I learned, connected and understood things in a world that was clearly "different." This became painfully true one day when a baby sitter found me talking to a stone wall, obviously deep in conversation with something or someone she did not see. Her reaction got bigger with each response, making me more aware of the "craziness" of what I was doing. "What are you doing, Shery?" Then "what ARE you doing?" And finally, "WHAT ARE YOU DOING?" By the end of her questioning, I had already learned that there was something "wrong" with me and that it was "bad."

This sense of myself also contributed to thinking that the abuse and violence I had been experiencing was my fault. I began to think being abused was pretty normal, as I was continuously being told, "it's for your own good," "it's your fault," or finally, "you must be crazy, that never happened." The abuse then continued on and on and there was no language for it. More and more it supported the "something wrong with me" theory. In conversations with other people, I had learned to "act as if ", pretending to be present, which continued to support and make me feel "other-than."

Finally I became overwhelmed and my ability to "act as if" no longer worked. I ended up speaking a language that others didn't understand, running around in the winter without socks or shoes, shaking and stuttering uncontrollably, or not being able to speak for days on end. Now the whole community told me I was crazy. I landed in the local psychiatric unit, locked up, in seclusion (with only a tiny observation window) and drugged when I started to shake. They told me I "had" something called schizophrenia. They never asked what had happened, nor heard my "story." Thorazine, at the time, was the drug of choice and it stopped *any* ability I'd had before to think, feel, participate in healthy relationships, or think about my experience in new ways.

My relationships with my fellow "patients" were based on what they had learned in the hospital. Their stories were stories of illness. From them I learned how to "cheek" my medications, hoard razor blades and sharp glass, and how to survive an EEG. After the many months I spent there, and after a series of shock treatments that erased most of my memory, I had learned to live the life of a mental patient. I had learned that I "had" something that others didn't, and then I learned how to hide it in the arts. It was somewhat easier being "crazy" as a poet and musician!

What would have been different about this story if talking to chipmunks had been seen as "normal"?

_____

_____

_____

_____

Can you remember the first time you felt different from others? Is so, describe it here.

_____

_____

_____

_____

How do you think that's affected the way you see yourself?

_____

_____

_____

_____

How has it affected your relationships?

_____

_____

_____

Many of us learned about our "otherness" or "differentness" in our first contact with the mental health system. This is due to the fact that the very first conversation we have when we come into the system involves an assessment. Once we've been assigned a diagnosis, we talk about treatment for "it." We've then lost who we are to a generic label. We begin to think about all of our experiences in relationship to illness: tough feelings as depression, excited feelings as mania, etc. No matter what we are feeling, when we talk about our feelings using this language, the conversation can only go in one direction. Pretty soon everything we do, think, and say runs through the "mental patient" filter.

Being a "mental patient" can become a full time job and once we've taken it on, we really are tied into the system. Our finances, housing, support, and job opportunities are dependent on our job as a "mental patient". (Prescott, 2002).

Just for fun think about the job of being a "mental patient:"

What is the job description?

_____

_____

_____

_____

Who assigns the job/role?

_____

_____

Who evaluates mental patients?

_____

_____

_____

What does it pay? What are the benefits?

_____

_____

_____

What are the drawbacks?

_____

_____

_____

What happens if you quit?

_____

_____

_____

This job becomes who we are and how we relate. Even in peer centers I've heard people refer to members as "the clients," "the consumers"…even "those people." I've heard conversations start with, "We're a Peer Support center/group that provides help for people with mental illness," rather than saying "We are a Peer Support center where people come to learn new ways of doing and being and to work on developing meaningful relationships".

When we start off the conversation in the first way, what do you think new members will think about the kinds of relationships they are going to have?

_____

_____

_____

What are some of the dynamics that might occur in the group/program?

_____

_____

_____

In Peer Support we make our "first contact" a different conversation. It is not useful for us to continue to treat and be with each other as "mental patients". What if our first conversation was to explain that Peer Support is a place where people are changing their lives and their perceptions of themselves, and a place to come to be with people who are committed to growth? What if our first question for a new member was, "Tell me about the most recent experience you've had doing something you didn't think you could do?"

What would the conversation be like? What would happen to people's relationships and future conversations?

_____

_____

_____

How would that change the task and the purpose of Peer Support?

_____

_____

To really enhance these conversations it is important to think about the core values we want to embody in our programs. Values are standards and beliefs that drive all of our assumptions, reactions, behaviors, and interactions.

In recent years as a recovery focus has come to the forefront in the mental health field, it has become clear that there are certain values and ethics that must guide all recovery work, including WRAP and Peer Support. They include the following:

1) **Hope**—Hope is the spark of life. A commonly held belief has been that those of us who experience certain kinds of "symptoms" can never get well, and will probably worsen over time. We have learned that this is not true—that we can and do get well and go on to do the things we want to do with our lives. Negative prognoses hinder recovery. We need to give each other messages of hope and insist that our supporters do the same.

2) **Self determination, personal responsibility, empowerment and self advocacy**—these words all remind us that while we may reach out to others for guidance and support, our recovery is "up to us". In the past others have tried to take away our control over our lives. Now we know that we have to take back that control, doing what we want to do the way we want to do it, and move forward. This is expanded when we think about mutual responsibility, where everyone works together towards and for the "life" of the program

3) **Treating each other as equals with dignity, compassion, mutual respect and unconditional high regard**—We need to insist on being treated well by those with whom we associate and to avoid people who treat us badly. This also means being direct and honest with each other in Peer Support.

4) **Unconditional acceptance of each person as they are: unique, special individuals, including acceptance of diversity with relation to cultural, ethnic, religious, racial, gender, age, disability and sexual preference issues**—There is no room for judgments or bigotry in this important work. Individual differences are valued as we move forward together.

5) **"No-limits" to recovery**—No one, no matter how highly educated, can accurately foretell the course of our lives. We determine our own course and our own goals, and work toward them as we wish, in spite of objections from others who may see our goals as unattainable.

6) **Choices and options, not final answers**—There are many roads we can take. It is up to us to choose our own road, making course corrections as we choose to do so.

7) **Voluntary participation**—Working towards one's recovery is a personal decision. No one else can make that decision for us.

8) **Personal expertise**—We are the experts on ourselves. No one else knows as much

about us as we do, but we must also be held accountable for practicing the values of Peer Support and WRAP.

9) **Clinical, medical and diagnostic language is discouraged**—Clinical language and diagnoses have often limited our understandings and possibilities. It is not necessary, and is not desirable, to use this language when working on recovery.

10) **Focus on working together to increase mutual understanding, knowledge and promote wellness**—Those of us who have had difficult feelings and behaviors learn various recovery options from each other and support each other as we work toward recovery.

11) **Adaptable to anyone's personal philosophy**—the flexibility of these options have been found to work for everyone, regardless of their personal belief system, ethnic or cultural background.

12) **Emphasis on strategies that are simple and safe for anyone and away from strategies that may have harmful effects**—Many "treatments" that were administered "in our best interest" have left us with horrible long term effects like post traumatic stress disorder, tardives dyskinesia, loss of memory, excess weight and diabetes. Peer Support and WRAP focus attention on safe, free strategies that promote health and well-being.

13) **Normalize responses**—In the past our responses to difficult situations have been seen as "abnormal" when they were actually normal responses to difficult circumstances. Peer Support and WRAP validate these responses and support us as we work with and through them.

14) **Focus on strengths and away from perceived deficits**—In the past many of us have been evaluated based on what others perceived as our deficiencies. In WRAP and Peer Support, the focus is on using our strengths to work through adversity, create change and make our lives the way we want them to be.

15) **The body of knowledge is always expanding and is infinite**—While some factions of the mental health field are using dated quantitative research findings to justify imposition of long term programs, WRAP and Peer Support programs will grow and change according to the needs of the people who use them and are most affected by them, through a process of on-going assessment and course correction.

Other values of Peer Support and WRAP include:

- Empathy *and* accountability
- Having fun
- Valuing community
- Taking care of yourself

- Not using symptoms as an excuse for bad behavior
- Learning to work through conflict
- Giving and receiving critical feedback
- Mutual validation
- Confidentiality

If you can think of other values and ethics that you feel should guide this work, list them here.

_____

_____

_____

The following experience made me even more aware of why stated values are so important.

> A woman had been coming to our peer center for some time. One of the values that she stressed was that everyone must share responsibility for the maintenance and growth of the program. However, on one particular occasion she didn't show up for work. She did, however, call our warm line to say that she wasn't feeling too well but didn't need any help. The next call was a little more dramatic. She called and said she was going out to buy some alcohol but that we shouldn't worry. Finally she called and said that she thought she might take some extra medication with the alcohol but once again told us not to check up on her. About that time, others were getting scared and I was getting frustrated. I called her and asked if we could talk. There was some hesitation but she invited me to her house. We talked at length about what was happening (the calls and the request for no help), and wondered together how her actions fit with the kind of mutually responsible relationships we were trying to create. After some time her voice got pretty quiet and she said, "You're right, I guess I wasn't sure that anyone really cared, and this was a way for me to find out." For me (and I think for the rest of the center) that was a turning point. We started to get really good at reflecting on our ability to practice values, rather than being critical of each other's behavior. This contributed to an environment where people became more self-reflective, and opened us up to putting our values into action.

We also come to peer programs with our own personal values and beliefs. _Culture_ is a useful concept for helping us understand not only how we have learned to make meaning of our personal experience, but also how our interaction with the mental health system has contributed to our sense of culture. If we become more aware of how our experiences have formed us, we have a much greater chance of creating something different.

Chapter 3
Culture & Peer Support

What is culture?

Generally, the aspects of culture that we think about are ethnicity, religion, race, and perhaps geographic. Rarely do we stop to think about the way our culture has influenced most of our beliefs and behaviors. Culture is not just the customs of the country that you come from, but the beliefs, rituals, roles, kinds of information you get, and messages about who you are. It is how you define yourself and how you see the world. Everyone gets different messages. Some of the messages we may have gotten are, "an eye for an eye," "children should be seen and not heard," "boys don't cry," "don't cry over spilt milk," etc.

What were the messages you got, for example, about conflict?

_____

_____

_____

_____

Mental health also has its own culture but it has been interpreted in a variety of ways in different countries. For example, when someone in Japan has a headache they might be referring to what we call depression. In other cultures, what we may call a psychotic break may be interpreted as a spiritual journey. In western culture we've been told that mental illness is a biological brain disorder that makes us act in certain ways. Others say there is no such thing as mental illness.

What are your some of your beliefs about mental illness?

_____

_____

_____

_____

Where and how did you learn those beliefs?

_____

_____

_____

_____

Along the way, we also learned how to act when we weren't feeling well, based on the kind of "help" responses we got. These responses also taught us a lot about what help meant.

What are some of the behaviors you developed when you were "sick" (e.g. complaining always gets results; grin and bear it; etc.)?

_____

_____

_____

_____

What are some of the things you learned about "help" (always listen to the doctor; do things for people until they're all better; treat people like children; only got help in dire emergencies; etc.)?

_____

_____

_____

_____

One day when I went to a meeting at the local community mental health center, I was really affected by what I saw. There on the smoking porch were many of the members of our peer program. They were waiting to get their medications and their social security check. People kept their heads down, shuffled around and looked rather defeated. What limited conversation they did have focused almost exclusively on illness. People talked about their various crises, need for appointments, why they needed more money from their payee, etc. Maybe you're thinking that this would not be an unusual conversation for a mental health center and it probably isn't. The interesting thing was that these very same people had a completely different kind of conversation on the peer center smoking porch. It was always energetic and lively. People talked about their friends and their weekends, they talked about politics and what should happen at the peer center. It was like night and day. This phenomenon led me to believe that not only do we have our own cultural experience but that we shape how we behave to fit the way we think others perceive us and to the environment we're in.

In the Peer Support movement our stories have also created a culture. This culture is different from traditional mental health in that we relate to one another based on shared experiences. We can be helpful to each other because we "get it." Peer Support culture doesn't use medical language. For example, people are not patients, their diagnosis is not important, and we don't do assessment and evaluation. Peer Support operates on shared/negotiated decision-making and it is a "learning" rather than a "treatment" environment.

But sometimes when there is conflict or stress in our programs or groups, we find ourselves acting just like people in the worst kind of treatment environments. We assume that we are not "expert" enough to handle a situation, we tell each other to "Get over it," or we tell each other what to do.

What happens in your peer program or group when the going gets rough?

_____

_____

_____

It is important to notice how our beliefs and ideas affect how we do Peer Support. If we don't pay attention, we may end up doing to each other what's been done to us, and we may behave in old ways to get what we need. If we can learn to stand back from our own perspective and remember that we've all had different messages about illness and help, we'll find that we can build more trusting, healing, and respectful relationships.

Understanding "the House"

I've often used "the house" as a way of thinking about our personal culture and how each of us has learned to see the world, and also to help us remember that people are complex, unique, and forever changing. Not only do we speak from various "rooms" on the inside of our house, we may also change our "story" based on whom we're talking to.

Each of us lives within a house. It has an outside that others see and an inside no one else can see or fully know. Its basic framework is the physical, emotional and spiritual self that we are born with. Over the years, many changes are made to our house—both inside and outside. Its rooms become "decorated" by all the messages and experiences we've had. For example, if early in life we are adored, talked to, held and told that we are the most wonderful person on earth, our house might include plush rugs, attractive furniture and a fireplace. If an important person then comes into our life and gives us negative messages, the interior of our house changes. Often negative messages and fears are put in our basement or closet where dark secrets are kept. More positive messages create upstairs rooms with windows and doors where it is sunnier, where relationships are more transparent, and communication goes back and forth. Messages of "otherness" might create an attic. Needless to say, the view from the basement is different than the view from the attic and our perspective changes as we move from room to room.

For example: If I'm in my basement, and I'm looking out a window, how will my location affect what I see?

_____

_____

_____

_____

If I'm upstairs in a sunny, warm room, how will that location affect what I see out the window?

_____

_____

_____

_____

If my "house" has lots of dark, tiny rooms and not much light, how will that affect what I see outside?

_____

_____

_____

_____

Or if my "house" is full of light with not much dark, how will that affect my view?

_____

_____

_____

_____

The houses in the neighborhood look alike on the outside. We really can't see their insides, but because they look similar, we think we know what they might look like. Then, when we talk to a person, we sometimes make the mistake of "over-relating." We say: "I know what you mean, I've had the exact same experience." This is one of the mistakes often found in Peer Support groups where we over-identify and keep relating to each other from the "patient" role.

For a long time my house seemed to have nothing but a big basement. Although people thought I was upstairs, those rooms just offered the appearance of being lived in. As I got clearer about the way I had learned to see the world and to relate to others, I began to move out of the basement, into the living room and finally out to the front porch.

How would you describe the inside of your "house?"

_____

_____

_____

_____

What room do you spend the most time in? How has that changed over time?

_____

_____

_____

_____

Why do you think that has changed?

_____

_____

_____

_____

The Context of "Story:"

In lots of ways we also talk about ourselves based on what we think the listener assumes about us. Because we've spent a lot of time in the mental health system, we have learned to tell many people our "mental illness story". We assume that it's what people see when they look at us. Often when we start working, we tell our "work story" and say things like, "I used to be a 'consumer' but now I'm staff."

Why do you think we might tell a "staff" kind of story instead of a "consumer" kind of story?

_____

_____

_____

_____

What kind of story do you tell when you're talking to your doctor (e.g. "My symptoms are under control" story)?

_____

_____

_____

_____

What kind of story do you tell when you're talking to your mother (e.g. an "Everything's fine" story)?

_____

_____

_____

What kind of story do you tell when you are talking to your friend (e.g. an "I'm feeling great, let's go to the park" story.)?

_____

_____

_____

_____

We learn to tell our stories based on who's listening, how much we trust them, what impact we want to have, and our assumptions about the way they think.

Chapter 4
Language and the Power of Words

Some say that language is the most powerful tool we have. We can knock down, build up, categorize and even control the direction of the whole conversation just by the language we use. While some language is useful in terms of description, it may also be filled with negative images and used to "pigeon-hole" us or "keep us in our place". In mental health we have a language that someone created to define and describe us as a group. Some of the words have even become standard in <u>our</u> conversations!

Exercise: Look at the following words and quickly let an image come into your head. Write down what you see.

- Chronic _____
- Consumer _____
- De-compensate _____
- Low-functioning_____
- Schizophrenic _____
- Borderline _____

How do these words make you feel about yourself? About others?

_____
_____
_____
_____

Choosing Words

Mental health language	Regular people language
Chronic	In recovery
Symptoms	Experiences
"High/low functioning"	"Having a good/bad day"
Manipulative	Strategic
"My client"	People I work with
Referred to by diagnosis	Person
"The mentally ill"	People
Non-compliant	Not in agreement with me

Mental health language	Regular people language
Treatment resistant	Considering other options
Safety	Feeling supported enough to try new things
Decompensate	Having a bad day

Think about some of the traps in the following sentences and re-write them in a way that might better represent a Peer Support perspective.

🐝 "The consumers in my program are unmotivated."
Instead I could say _____

🐝 "Maybe I should call the crisis line for you…"
Instead I could say _____

🐝 "Staff here are more recovered than members."
Instead I could say _____

🐝 "She's fragile/in crisis."
Instead I could say _____

🐝 "Staff should have good boundaries and never give out their home phone numbers."
Instead I could say _____

🐝 "No one ever wants to help me."
Instead I could say_____

🐝 "We don't take calls regarding suicidal feelings, call Crisis."
Instead I could say_____

Some possible responses:

🐝 People here have been taught to have low expectations.

🐝 How can I support you in doing what you need to do?

🐝 We're all working on our recovery and we all have good and bad days.

🐝 She has survived a lot and will get through this tough time.

🐝 It is good to figure out where and when to set limits.

🐝 I feel pretty isolated.

🐝 I'm a little scared about what's going on for you, how can we figure this out together?

Chapter 5
Listening Differently

Really listening to how others communicate offers us a broader, deeper understanding of them. It allows us to have a better idea of the layout and history of our respective "houses". When we listen with an understanding of how our cultures have influenced us, we are better able to help each other get out of rooms we're stuck in, begin to explore the rest of the house, and then help each other remodel.

How do you know when you're really listening?

_____

_____

_____

What gets in the way of really listening?

_____

_____

_____

How do you know when someone's really listening to you?

_____

_____

_____

What makes you feel really heard and validated?

_____

_____

_____

All too often we listen based on the way our house got built! It's amazing what happens when we make assumptions about each other and then listen through the lens of those assumptions. Even when we think we're really listening with compassion and empathy, we get in trouble if we assume too much.

One day a man came to the center who clearly hadn't bathed in a number of days, maybe weeks. When people at the center asked him to go home and bathe, he started talking about the shower emitting poisonous gas. People were getting frustrated and giving him bars of soap, but he wasn't interested and he was getting more and more distracted. Members kept commenting to each other that he was becoming delusional and "getting worse." They wanted to throw him out until he took a shower. Finally I sat down with him and said, "Seems like when people talk about bathing, you get really scared." He started talking about the poisonous gas and started to get louder. I said that it must be terrifying, no wonder he didn't want to shower. I told him that I used to be afraid of taking baths because I'd been abused there. He quieted down and his eyes welled up and he said that his father would punish him by coming in the bathroom when he was in the shower and turn up the temperature to scald him. It was punishment for wasting water.

Really listening helps us understand the bigger picture. Some listening skills that are important to Peer Support include:

Pay attention (to words, body language, feelings, etc.)

This might be the most obvious **and** the most difficult skill to master. Paying attention requires us to be fully present, not distracted, not "in our heads," not thinking about how we're going to respond. It means being fully available to the other person's experience of the inside of their house.

Provide validation ("That sounds tough. You must be really strong to..." "After what you've been through, no wonder you feel angry/sad/afraid.")

Once we've really listened to the story of the other person, we should acknowledge their experience. This means responding from the heart, adding something so they know we've really seen and heard them. I've heard this described as responding in such a way that they other person "feels us feeling what they're saying" (Miller & Stiver, 1997).

Reflection of feelings ("That must make you feel really sad...")

We often forget that at least half of what others are trying to say to us is not being communicated with words. If we're not listening for feelings we may misread the situation. For example someone might be telling us that their landlord is making them get rid of their cat. We assume they're mad but we need to ask...maybe they're afraid, confused, sad, etc. We won't know unless we say what we think they might be feeling. Making assumptions gets us into trouble.

Say back in your words what you think you're hearing

In order to make sure we're getting the gist of what they're saying, we can say back in our own words what we think they're saying. Sometimes language and emotions are hard to read. For example, if someone tells us that they are being "encouraged" to increase their medication at a time when they've been thinking about decreasing it, you might say, "Are you saying that you feel misunderstood?"

Listen with an ear for role

Sometimes we've gotten stuck in being "good patients". "Good patients" do what they are told, don't question the doctor, believe they need to be taken care of, etc. We may not be familiar with other ways of thinking about our experiences and our lives. This role has been compounded by discrimination, stigma, poverty, lack of resources and someone else defining our experience (e.g., you are sick; these are symptoms of a mental illness; you need to be taken care of). We have been taught to believe that help goes one direction only. "You're the helper, I'm the patient." Understand that this is how their house got built and recognize that it may be the only role that person knows right now.

Ask questions (learn more about the inside of their house)

Good questions are the key to opening up the story and more fully appreciating what the other person's experience has been. What would help us understand their perspective? How will we get a sense of the "big picture?" Notice with them what we're seeing and hearing. How will we help them see how they might have gotten where they are?

For example:

"I wonder how you decided to …"

"Can you help me understand why that's meaningful for you?"

"Have you ever wondered how you learned to think that way?"

Be aware of bias in your language

If we're using language the other person doesn't understand or trying to force our language on them, they may tend to feel disrespected and stop being willing to share. If we start with their language, we can gradually throw in ours. In other words, if they're talking about their mental illness, we shouldn't start by saying that we don't believe in mental illness. Ask the person what mental illness means to them. For example: someone says they're feeling unsafe. What does safety mean to them, look like, feel like? Is safety the same as protection, relinquishing responsibility, or is safety a trusting environment in which to try new things? If someone says, "I'm a schizophrenic," we might ask how they learned that? How did they think/talk about their experience before they were diagnosed?

Be authentic

In Peer Support we can help each other by beginning to explore some of the roles that have kept us stuck, offering each other new information and most importantly, creating a mutually responsible relationship. This means being honest and direct about what we can and can't do as well as what makes us really uncomfortable. Rather than trying to control the situation, it is important to say how we feel, say what we see, and then negotiate something that works for both of us. We are not responsible for taking care of anyone. We are only responsible for being as honest, open, and present as we can be.

Share relevant personal stories to build a connection

("I once had a similar experience, is it anything like that?")

This is where we can begin to see if their experience is anything like ours. It's a great time to think together about what it means and offer some things we may have learned. This is not a time for advice unless the person asks for it, and even then, keep it to a minimum. For example: A person comes to us and says that they're feeling lousy from their medications but afraid to tell their psychiatrist. Rather than telling them what we think they should do, we might say, "Boy, there was a time when I was feeling tired all the time from my medications, I couldn't get anything done. At that time I was a little afraid of my psychiatrist because he'd hospitalized me in the past, but I realized that not saying anything kept me in kind of a victim role…"

Maintain mutual responsibility

Even in Peer Support we sometimes find ourselves stuck in being just the "helper" or the "helped." We start to think the people in our programs are fragile and need to be taken care of. We stop saying what we think, not wanting to risk saying the "wrong thing," or "setting someone off." Creating a mutually responsible relationship means both people are committed to talking through differences, sharing feelings and, to some extent, supporting each other. For example, when someone says over and over that they are sick of living, we might say; "I understand that you feel that way often. I guess I'm not sure what it is that you want me to do. I feel a little frustrated and a little scared." (Note: this is much more helpful than calling the police.) Another common example is the assumption that "staff" shouldn't ask members for support, worrying that it "might be too much for them." When this happens, members start to feel like "clients" or "patients". This can become a great time to reflect on assumptions as a group.

Build a direction together ("Maybe we could try…")

After sharing experiences with each other it becomes easier to figure out how our combined experience and knowledge will help with direction or problem solving. When trust and hope are created in a relationship it's amazing how "the power of two" can contribute to both people trying new things that might have been too scary to try alone. This has been defined as mutual empowerment: "a relationship that provides for both people a feeling of zest, it feels like an increase, not a decrease, in vitality, aliveness, energy. This increases courage or the ability to try out new thoughts and feelings on the other person" (Miller & Stiver, 1997).

What would you do if…

A peer came to you and was telling you about a situation similar to one you had last week. You're late for an appointment and dying to just move things along and tell the person what to do…

_____

_____

_____

One of your colleagues is constantly saying clinical words ("she's bi-polar," "that person is really low-functioning," etc.)

_____

_____

_____

_____

What would you say if you thought the other person was about to make a "bad" decision?

_____

_____

_____

_____

Key points:

There are many versions of the same story

We are only hearing one version of the story, because people tell their stories in certain ways based on who's listening. Sometimes they even have the desire to impress, to shock, or to distance themselves. It's important to remember that we're hearing the story based on our relationship with them (e.g., friend, relative, clinician etc.), and which "room of the house" they're in.

What we contribute influences the direction of the story

We ask certain questions based on the way *we're* hearing the story being told. The questions we ask, and how we ask them, change the story. For example, someone is telling you about how rough their weekend was and you ask if they've taken their medications. That will usually end the conversation. What could you say instead that might keep the conversation going, and that would be helpful to both of you?

Paying attention takes work and awareness

We stop listening for any number of reasons without even realizing it. Maybe we're hungry or tired or thinking about a similar experience. We need to remember to bring ourselves back to full presence when we find we've drifted. If you just can't listen because you are too tired, too hungry or have another appointment, let the other person know, and try to set up another time to get together.

What works for us may not work for another person

We often make judgments about other people's decisions based on our own experience. If we find ourselves thinking or even implying "Well, that's a stupid decision," stop, go back and ask questions that help clarify. Remember, people make decisions based on the inside of *their* house, not yours.

Coaching

Recently I've (Shery) started working with a personal coach and have realized the value of good listening, excellent questions, and a framework different than mental health. I remember the first conversation I had with my coach when I described my life situation (all the problems), expecting her to offer me better skills with which to manage. Her responses to questions didn't seem to relate to coping skills. All of a sudden I realized that we weren't focusing on problems at all, we were focusing on moments of joy (a concept I hadn't particularly associated with my life). We were talking about skills to create a whole new way of being, rather than skills that would simply deal with what was. As I practiced and put energy into "a vision," I realized how habitual my patterns of "coping with problems" had become and I realized that it would take practice and discipline AND support to enhance and build upon joy. Friends have now started to notice that I am more energetic, more awake, and are wondering how I made this shift.

The skills of coaching are very similar to the skills of Peer Support. If you've never gotten personal coaching, give it a try. When you've gotten hooked, you'll see the immediate possible applications for Peer Support programs and groups. It is tremendously important that we (as an alternative system) continue to look to other disciplines for tools that will be helpful.

Following is a definition of personal coaching offered to me by my coach (Buell, 2003).

> Coaching helps people produce extraordinary results in their lives, careers, businesses or organizations. The coaching relationship is based on the premise that you are the expert in your life and work, and that every one of us is creative, resourceful and whole.

> The purpose of coaching is to bridge the gap between where you are and where you want to be, whether it is in health, relationships, finances, career or any other area.

> Coaching is about action. The coach's responsibility is to discover, clarify, and align with what you want to achieve, to encourage self-discovery, to elicit self-generated solutions and strategies, and to hold you responsible and accountable. It is to challenge you (and support you in the process) to go beyond where you would normally stop. A coach helps you tap into your greatness.

> Active listening, powerful questions, curiosity, intuition and reflecting back are but a few of the skills coaches use to foster an interaction that creates clarity and action.

Coaching accelerates progress by providing greater focus and awareness of choice.

Coaching concentrates on where you are now and what you are willing to do to get where you want to be in the future, recognizing that results area matter of your intentions, choices and actions, supported by the coach's efforts and application of the coaching process.

The values and skills used in life coaching are the just what we need in Peer Support.

Chapter 6

What is Trauma-Informed Peer Support & Why is it Important?

Trauma informed Peer Support is based on understanding who people have become because of what they've been through. It helps us to identify the real, underlying problems or original trauma. Trauma informed Peer Support helps us understand people's stories, actions and relational skills with a greater sensitivity. Traditional services are beginning to assess people for histories of trauma and abuse. Even so, people utilizing these services are still being told that they are the ones with a "mental illness," not the person or people who hurt them.

Studies show that about 90% of the people that come through the mental health system have experienced trauma and abuse. Some of these include witnessing violence, childhood neglect, natural disasters, war related phenomena, sexual assault or rape (childhood or adult), physical assault, multiple losses, and even mental health "treatment." Judith Herman (1992) describes traumatic events as ones in which:

- The victims are rendered helpless by overwhelming force.
- There are threats to life or bodily integrity, or a close personal encounter with violence and death.
- Our sense of control, connection and meaning are disrupted.
- People are confronted with the extremities of helplessness and terror, and evoke the responses of catastrophe.

Unfortunately many people in the mental health system have been treated with no regard to the effects of these events.

In Peer Support we start with the assumption that our perceptions, how we interact with one another, and how we define our experience, have been significantly influenced by the particular trauma, abuse and other experiences of our lives. Trauma we have experienced shows up in our behaviors (self-injury, addictions), in our physical body (high pain threshold, weight issues), in the way we think about things (self hate, paranoia, delusions), in our emotions (shame, depression), and even in our spiritual lives (disconnection). Sometimes responses that appear dangerous may actually feel safer to us because of our past experience. For example, self-harm may feel safer than expressing our anger.

Because these responses have often been treated as symptoms of mental illness, we have learned to believe that strong or difficult feelings are dangerous and need treatment. This then leads to a sense of "learned helplessness," which we talked about earlier. When we see our own feelings and responses as signs of "mental illness," we may think that they are out of our control. As we learn more about our responses through WRAP and Peer Support, we realize we have many options. We learn to use the options that fit with what we want our lives to be like.

What would have happened to our "symptoms" if right from the start, people asked us, "What happened to you?" rather than asking, "What's wrong with you?" (Bloom, 1997)

_____

_____

_____

_____

What if they had told us that we are not the problem: the abuse was the problem? What would have changed about our assumptions, beliefs, and behaviors?

_____

_____

_____

_____

What happens for you when you have strong [difficult] feelings?

_____

_____

_____

_____

What happens to your relationships?

_____

_____

_____

_____

Sarah had been a recipient of mental health services for most of her life. She had been diagnosed with bipolar disorder and because of her history she was told to expect periodic episodes of mania. She was so accustomed to this schedule that she virtually prepared herself for hospitalization every year. This year, at the beginning of August, she came to our peer center. She described not sleeping, racing thoughts, images of death and blood, and an urgency about running into the woods with a knife. Rather than calling her case manager, I talked with her about having often felt like this as well, and told her how terrified I had been. We talked a lot about our images of death and blood and shared related experiences. We both talked about histories of past violence. She finally told me the story of an August when she had been held against her will and violently abused. When she had finally been released she ran through the woods for a long time, not knowing where she was or what she should do. Many years later, just before August, when she finally brought it up to her case manager, she was told to put the past behind her. That's exactly what she did, always one step behind her. Out of her sight but not out of her experience.

The day we met, we put both our pasts into the conversation. We shared strategies and ideas. Mostly we built a relationship that was not based on assessment but rather on shared truths and mutual empathy. Each year since then, Sarah has asked people to "wrap around" her in August. She talks to people and they talk to her. Her experience is not named, it is witnessed. She no longer has delusions, she has strong feelings. She doesn't see herself as out of control but rather in great pain. This pain now has meaning for her. It is her history and her experience and she has begun to transform it. She now helps others develop plans and strategies to move through crises differently, or even to prevent them all together (Mead & Hilton 2003).

Peer Support offers us the perfect opportunity to question how we have come to understand our experiences. Rather than thinking of our feelings, behaviors, and thoughts as symptoms, we can start to normalize them and think about the context in which they developed. Instead of evaluating or assessing each other's "safety," we can bear witness and think about how we'll work together to make the world a safer place for everyone. By sharing our stories with one another we can start to break down the isolation and shame that has kept us disconnected. In doing these things we can create a whole new language and interpretation for what used to be named for us.

Allow people to name their own experience

We have often learned how to understand the effects of trauma as seen through a medical lens. We have been called Borderlines (with no fondness), hysterical, high maintenance, and any number of other negative terms. We have started to view ourselves in the ways we've been viewed (sick, symptomatic, mentally ill). It is powerful to think we can help each other re-name our experiences. When we understand that something has been done to us rather than that something is wrong with us, we begin to re-think who we have become and what we have survive. And what we will need to do to heal.

How has your experience been explained to you?

_____

_____

_____

_____

_____

_____

_____

How did that make you feel about yourself?

_____

_____

_____

_____

_____

How do you think that might affect the way you "help" others?

_____

_____

_____

_____

_____

What would have been more helpful?

_____

_____

_____

_____

_____

Witness rather than fix

It is incredibly powerful when we learn that we are not the only ones who struggle with the things we struggle with. It's also powerful to share the strengths we have developed for moving through those struggles. When we hear others' stories and when we see the healing they've done, it offers us hope and possibilities. And it reminds us that no two people's experiences are exactly the same. As we work together, remember that we are there not to compare or assess, but rather to learn together what a powerful effect trauma has had on our lives.

What does it feel like for you when you've thought you were "the only one" and then someone else shares a similar experience?

_____

_____

_____

_____

How has it felt to you when someone has really listened, validated your experiences and cared?

_____

_____

_____

Pay attention to power and roles we fall into

It is powerful to tell our stories to people who will simply witness, rather than assess, evaluate and judge us, especially if we have never been heard before. Sometimes, however, rather than building real connection, we find ourselves feeling defensive, competitive, powerless, scared, "less than," etc. We fall into roles in which communication tends to break down. I tell you the story of my healing and you tell me that's nothing compared to yours. I think you don't care about me and start to get angry. We get into a power struggle and we no longer are really listening to each other. Paying attention to these dynamics will allow us to name them and change them (more on that later).

How might you tell your story differently if you know that someone is doing an assessment or an evaluation on you?

_____

_____

_____

_____

What happens for you when someone tells you that "your experience is nothing" compared to theirs?

_____

_____

_____

_____

Negotiate reality

Often others have decided for us what is real and what is a delusion. This is not helpful. What we can do is offer our own reality while absolutely believing that the other person is experiencing theirs. In order to grow in relationship we must negotiate how we'll both proceed from that point. For example: A friend called me when he was having a tough time. He was clearly panicked and said that the FBI had bugged his apartment. He was also worried that if he left, they would follow him. That experience was very real for him. I knew it wouldn't be useful or respectful to tell him not to worry, that it was not really happening. Instead I asked him what we could do together to help him feel less afraid. I shared a story about a fear I'd often had of people reading my mind. I told him that this fear had gotten easier to deal with after remembering someone reading my diary and then being hospitalized. He said that his father had been a judge and that he'd felt like every move he made was being scrutinized. Slowly but surely he sounded sad rather than panicked. We talked about helping each other with old feelings and responses.

What happens for you when you experience something in a really powerful way and then someone says, "You shouldn't feel that way," "That's not really happening," "You must be getting sick again"?

_____

_____

_____

_____

Look for the larger context in which all our experiences relate

When we've been told that our experiences are signs of mental illness, when we've heard again and again that we are fragile, manipulative, and/or symptomatic, we stop trying. We think we have no control over our "illness" and we believe that we need to be taken care of. In Peer Support we can challenge this thinking. How can we be fragile if we've survived what we've survived? Why do people always say our behavior is manipulative when it's what has kept us safe? Maybe what we're experiencing are just "big feelings". Anyone would feel that way if they'd been through what we've been through.

How is it for you when you think of all your feelings as signs of mental illness?

_____

_____

_____

_____

Build a connection

Relationships have been difficult for many of us because of all the hidden and not so hidden abuse and dishonesty in our lives. It's up to us to model relationships that work for both people. This means constantly negotiating, maintaining an awareness of power imbalances, and being really honest and respectful.

Sometimes it's not so easy to figure out what to say when someone is having a difficult time. We tend to worry that if we say the wrong think something bad will happen, and so we say nothing. We must maintain connection by being honest, empathic, and authentic.

Language that helps:

- "That must feel horrible."
- "Although I don't totally know what you went/are going through, I've had similar reactions."
- "Help me understand…"
- "What are we going to do?"
- "It's not okay with me if you scream at me. How can we talk about this so we both feel safe?
- "I get really scared/sad/angry when you…"
- "We may not see things exactly the same way, but I believe you!"

What else might you say?

_____

_____

_____

_____

Language that hurts:

- "It can't be that bad…"
- "You should just get over it."
- "You must be exaggerating."
- "You're triggering me."

What are some other things that people have said to you that weren't helpful?

_____

_____

_____

_____

Chapter 7
Trauma Re-enactment

No matter how safe and connected we feel with our peers, when the "going gets rough," we tend to fall into some of our old patterns and roles. This is when things can really break down. We find ourselves gossiping, getting secretive or bossy, falling into victim roles or sometimes simply disappearing.

This dynamic is not unique to peer centers. It happens in businesses, families, communities, and agencies, anywhere people spend time together. If we think about this in the context of "trauma-worldview," we might see this as re-enacting our abuse.

Trauma re-enactment means that when a current situation triggers feelings from an old traumatic event, we fall into behaviors and responses that were relevant to the original event, but are probably not relevant to what is currently happening. For example, when someone says something to me that makes me feel ashamed, my instinctual response is to become self-destructive, feel like I've done something really bad, and perhaps start to relate to the person as if he/she had tremendous power over me. In relationships, when either person feels triggered it may create disproportionate distrust, creating the tendency to move into victim/aggressor roles. When there is a situation that triggers a whole program or group, we see people forming cliques, abusing power, leaving the program, or simply becoming invisible.

> A program I work with recently hired several people who had previously been volunteers. These particular people were extremely well liked and also admired for their dedication, their ability to support others, and their leadership. After they were hired however, the dynamics in the program started to change. Where once there had been clear communication and mutual support, it seemed that now, no matter what the new workers did, people saw them as "bossy," "favored over others," and even "abusive." Cliques started to form and not-so-nice messages started going around the group. As the dynamics progressed, some people started to leave the community, while others said they were becoming "symptomatic." The new workers felt under-appreciated and attacked. They also didn't understand why taking more responsibility for making things happen got them into trouble. Finally it was suggested that everyone meet and talk through assumptions about power, paid positions, roles and responsibilities. Clearly, relationships didn't feel the same when some people were paid and others were volunteers (even if volunteering had been by choice). It was decided that a lot of assumptions had been unfounded, but also, that when some people are paid, there is a power difference. It needed to be talked about openly and honestly, rather than having people fall into old roles and ways of relating to discomfort and secrecy.

When trauma re-enactment does occur in a group or program, we may find ourselves in situations that are scary or tremendously frustrating; certainly not comfortable. We then often want to control the situation by taking power in whatever ways we've learned. For example, when someone says that they feel suicidal, we may hear a peer say, "You shouldn't feel that way," or "Maybe I should call your case manager". Unfortunately, this is how we get into making decisions <u>for</u> people instead of <u>with</u> them. We are afraid they "can't take care of themselves," or "can't make good decisions," and we think we must "take over". An awareness of this tendency helps us to stay authentic rather than controlling.

What happens for you when someone thinks they need to take care of you? Protect you?

_____

_____

_____

_____

What happens for you when a friend who says they'll go out with you doesn't show up?

_____

_____

_____

_____

When whole programs are stuck we may hear things like, "So and so should be kicked out," "Let staff decide," and maybe even "We're too sick to have our own program."

In these situations people fall into various roles in relation to the discomfort. Some of these roles include victim, hero, scapegoat, aggressor, peacemaker, blamer etc.

When there's conflict in your center/group, what is a role you're likely to fall into? Why?

_____

_____

_____

_____

A couple of years ago I was working with a program that was teaching recovery and Peer Support skills. It was a popular place to go and a place where most everyone participated and contributed. One day a man came in saying that he didn't like the lunch that was being prepared. He said that there was too much salt in it. Members started to defend the lunch but the situation escalated. The man got up and said that he'd make sure the program got shut down. Well, all of a sudden everyone scrambled into familiar roles. I saw one person get really angry, another person try to calm the situation down, several people get really quiet and "invisible," many people try to get the director to throw the man out, and the person preparing the lunch say that he never was good at cooking anyhow. A couple of weeks later, I came back and we did an analysis of people's roles and the power dynamics I had witnessed. People laughed as they saw themselves reliving their past and we talked about what the program might have done differently. Suggestions included asking the person with the complaint if he'd like to help make the lunch, asking what it was about the situation that made him so angry, referring to the values of shared responsibility, and even calling the man on his use of power, and calling each other on our less than responsible reactions.

To make Peer Support work, we persist, building mutual, respectful, adult relationships. We're willing to witness people's pain, but also to hold people accountable for their end of the relationship, and their part in making the program work. We challenge each other when we find ourselves in old roles and we name the power dynamics for what they are. Trauma re-enactment will never go away completely, but how we respond to it can make or break our program.

Chapter 8

Creating Mutually Responsible Relationships: Negotiating Power

Sometimes it's not so easy to be honest. We get scared that if we say the wrong thing, the other person will get mad at us, go away, or get their feelings hurt. It's even harder to be honest when the situation is frightening or conflictive, but it is then that we need to really work at staying present, authentic and responsible. This means being willing to hear and explore the other person's story, and also willing to say what you see, need and want. What too often happens in difficult situations is that when we get scared we use our power in whatever way was successful for us in the past. We yell, lie, use our position, become condescending, or even a little too "helpful."

Describe a time when you've used your power to get what you wanted. What did that do to the relationship?

_____

_____

_____

_____

Describe a time when power was taken from you. How did you respond?

_____

_____

_____

_____

When we are afraid or uncomfortable it is common to want to take control of the situation. I don't think I've yet been to a program where people don't sometimes fall into the role of "doing what's been done to them," when they're confronted with a difficult situation. But it is in these difficult situations that we must step back and think about whose need it is that we're trying to meet. Doing this helps separate out our discomfort from the situation and allows us to say what we need and want without making demands. This might be as simple as saying, "This is making me feel really uncomfortable right now, and I'm not sure how to respond."

Saying what we see, need and want after we've really heard the other person is crucial. This means being honest even when we're afraid of hurting the other person's feelings, making them mad, or worried that we'll push them "over the edge".

Exercises:

1) **What would you do if someone you were working with told you something uncomfortable and then said that they don't want you to tell anyone else?**

_____

_____

_____

_____

Sometimes being mutually responsible means negotiating some difficult issues. In this situation we might say, "I really want to hear what you have to say and I feel a little trapped when you tell me to keep secrets."

2) **How would you respond if someone said "You're not helping…my case manager wouldn't do things that way."**

_____

_____

_____

_____

It's hard not to get defensive. It's hard to want to "see inside someone's house" when they criticize you but we might say something like, "I wonder what you mean when you say, 'You don't help?' I feel a little hurt."

3) **What if someone were coming in and out of your program a lot, almost appearing to be "creating crises"?**

_____

_____

_____

_____

It's easy to be judgmental rather than mutually responsible. You might say, "I feel a little frustrated when it seems like you are coming in every day with another crisis. I wonder if you feel safer doing that?"

4) **What happens when a person says that more medication is the only way to get through the night, and you feel certain they're already over-medicated?**

_____

_____

_____

_____

Although we're tempted to argue for or against medication, it is not our "turf." We can advocate with someone with their doctor if they want us to, but we never make medication recommendations ourselves. You might say: "What is it about medications that you find helpful? I wonder if you've thought of other ways to get that kind of help?

What's different about this kind of help?

_____

_____

_____

_____

Patty was a woman who had been in psychiatric hospitals many times. Recently she had completed training to become a respite worker in our Peer Run Crisis Alternative. That training helped her understand her tendency to take on a victim role. She maintained this self-awareness until she was having a rough time. One day she came in to work and was very quiet. She said that she was feeling kind of low and needed to go to the hospital. I felt my judgments start to creep in but listened to her rationale. After a while I asked her to help me understand what the hospital actually meant for her. She said that they would take care of her when she didn't think she could take care of herself. I wondered if there was another way she could get what she needed to take care of herself. She didn't have any other solutions. Finally I said, "Patty, do you remember when we talked about roles we fall into when we're uncomfortable? What role would you say you might be in right now?" Well that did it, she got pretty mad at me and said clearly that I didn't understand and maybe this whole respite thing was pretty stupid anyway! About 20 minutes later she came back to the center and said, "Yeah, I was doing the victim role. When I feel bad, it feels like no one could possibly care. I feel unworthy, like there is nothing I could possibly do to be OK. I guess I've used the hospital as kind of an escape. Do you think maybe I could come into respite for a couple of days?" She stayed for the weekend and then returned as a respite worker the following week.

No matter what the situation is, before you react, think about your own discomfort and what that means. Think about the context that the other person/people have come from and consider the fact that their experience is their truth and reality. Be aware that growth happens only when people are first heard and validated. However, your context, your experience, and your needs are equally important and must be part of negotiating the situation. Staying open to different perspectives while holding your own is something that would benefit everyone in the world. In Peer Support we can model this strategy by continuing to explore the "inside of other people's houses," while re-modeling our own.

Some useful tips to remember:

- Use I statements…(e.g. "I feel scared when you…," "When you do 'x', I feel frustrated," "When I feel triggered, I…").
- Don't intentionally dig up past abuse.
- BELIEVE PEOPLE, even if their reality is different from your reality.
- Avoid "mental health" language: (e.g. tough feelings vs. symptoms, intensity vs. crisis, having a bad day vs. getting sick).
- Stay aware of some of the roles people tend to fall into when they're stressed.
- Share some of the things you've done to get through.
- Create HOPE and develop TRUST.
- Getting "unstuck" may mean learning to sit with discomfort.
- Learn to tolerate difficult situations.
- Stay present (not getting distracted by what you want to say, focusing on now rather than thinking about times in the past, etc.)
- Hold your beliefs while trying out new ones at the same time.
- Balance between "going away" and "getting overwhelmed" (staying present to the other person but listening to and respecting your own process/needs as well).
- Negotiate: remember, both people matter.
- If the relationship's not working for both people, it's not working!

Boundaries

What do you think of when you think about boundaries? Personally, I think of stone walls: something firm and not changing. In mental health, clinicians are taught that boundaries keep people in "appropriate" roles: the patient is the patient and the clinician is not. In Peer Support we don't have fixed roles with each other. Sometimes we are the listener, sometimes the listened to, and sometimes that even changes in one conversation! This gets confusing sometimes.

The language of limits has different implications than the language of boundaries. We set limits with people based on what both of our needs are at a given time. For some things we even come up with permanent limits. For example, I go to bed really early, so I ask people never to call me after 9 PM. This sets up a very different dynamic than saying that people can never call me at home. It also leaves room to change the limit based on a specific experience. If someone has called me every night for a week, I might say that I need them to call someone else for a while – that it's not working for me. On some weeks I might ask people not to call me at all.

What are some of your limits or boundaries?

_____

_____

_____

_____

What is your experience with setting limits with people? How did you learn to do it?

_____

_____

_____

_____

Is it sometimes hard to keep others from violating your boundaries? Why do you think that is?

_____

_____

_____

_____

Sometimes traditional mental health boundary policies become pretty tempting because they allow us to set an arbitrary line and not have to set individual, situational limits. For example we start telling people that workers don't ever give out their home number or we say that workers can't be recipients or guests. We start using boundaries to separate ourselves and then fall into the same power dynamics as a traditional helping relationship.

Michael and John were co-workers in a respite program. They were mutually supportive and were able to use their relationship to help each other work through tough times. One weekend, John was having an exceptionally difficult time and asked if he could come into the respite program. He was relieved when he found out that Michael was working that weekend. John's respite stay was really helpful and he returned to work the following week. As always he went to Michael at the end of the day to compare notes and to get some Peer Support. It hadn't been an easy transition. Michael was quite cold and said rather bluntly, "workers can't be friends with guests." John was crushed. When had this policy been set? How did that fit with Peer Support? At the community meeting, John asked if this new policy had been implemented during his respite stay. He was told that there was no such policy. When confronted, Michael told John that he had been afraid to do Peer Support with him now because he worried he might say the wrong thing.

Sometimes we may find ourselves in some pretty confusing situations. Some of them may even require policies for clarity. But most of the time it is best if we figure out what our limits are in a given situation, and then make our limits really clear to the people around us. This will not only be good modeling for people who have not learned to set limits, but also helps build trust.

Think about a situation where you set a limit with someone and it really helped the relationship in the long run. How did you negotiate it? How did that create greater safety for both of you?

_____

_____

_____

_____

_____

_____

_____

_____

_____

_____

_____

_____

_____

_____

_____

_____

_____

Chapter 9
Conflict

Conflict is something that most organizations struggle with and just about no one loves. Conflict happens when a difference of opinion becomes a problem between two people, a group, or even a whole program. Though it may be uncomfortable, working through conflict creates the potential for significant growth and deepening relationships.

Fully understanding this process, and being willing to make it part of your peer group or program's culture, will determine the quality, and perhaps, the life of your program.

How has conflict been handled in your peer group/program?

_____

_____

_____

_____

Let's look at a common example. Suppose there is one member who is consistently asking others for favors it seems like he's perfectly capable of doing for himself. We may start out with an attitude of, "Oh well, it's no big deal." But by about the third time he asks, we're getting frustrated and perhaps a little resentful. We start to talk about this member to each other in not so nice ways or we simply yell, "Do it yourself!"

What happened here? Our immediate reaction might be something like, "Well this guy was just being lazy and manipulative." But why did it seem like no big deal to begin with?

_____

_____

_____

_____

Because we've not asked why he's continuing to ask favors, we assume a whole lot. We make these assumptions based on our past experiences, and then, no matter what happens, we've already created a picture of the situation. What if, for example, someone continuously asking for favors triggers for us our experience with an alcoholic parent who was demanding and cruel? We might think, "Well, I'm an adult now and I'm not letting this guy walk all over me, too!"

What if this person has been asking for favors because he's been living in a group home and gets in trouble when he does things without asking?

_____

_____

_____

_____

Our mismatched interpretations have now created two conflicting realities that can't possibly both be true (or so we think). We get defensive about our position and lock in. But this could also be a time to explore one another's feelings and perceptions and then negotiate what will work best with both people.

What are some ways of doing this?

_____

_____

_____

_____

Before blowing a gasket or starting to gossip maybe we could say, "You've been asking me to do things for you a lot lately, and I'm beginning to feel pretty frustrated. Can you help me understand why you ask others to do things for you that you seem able to do yourself? Is there something else that you need that you're not asking for?"

This offers the member an opportunity to think about what's going on right now and without getting put on the defensive, he/she might say, "I'm sorry, I didn't realize people were getting frustrated. I just didn't want to do the wrong thing by doing it myself. I thought I might get into trouble."

Where might this conversation go from here?

_____

_____

_____

_____

What would have happened if we let more time pass and no one addressed the situation directly?

_____

_____

_____

_____

It is important to remember that everyone has a perception and a way of understanding and doing things based on something that's been real for them.

Can you think of a recent conflict you've been involved in where you let your assumptions drive what you did?

_____

_____

_____

_____

What happened?

_____

_____

_____

_____

When we experience conflict, the first thing we can do is to check out our "story." What do we believe these actions mean? Is it possible they could mean something different than that? How would we know? Making any assumptions that our perceptions are the "truth" will get us into trouble every time. Remember that most people don't do hurtful things intentionally. Whatever version the other person has is their "truth." Whatever the situation is, slow down, take a breath, get present, take a break, start with I statements (I feel frustrated when you…I'm feeling a little attacked, etc.). Do whatever it is that you need to do to remember that your assumptions are just that: your assumptions! When we are able to successfully work through conflict, our programs and groups help people to be better advocates, better friends, and better leaders.

Chapter 10
Evaluating our Efforts

Because these programs are attempting to apply a different approach to "help," it is critical that a forum is provided for on-going feedback and evaluation; a forum that supports our ability to evolve as a learning organization. This means that all participants in the program (peer workers, guests, peer members, and any administrative staff) must be able to critique each other through the lens of program values. It is important to set meetings where everyone knows ahead of time that this will be a time for offering critical feedback, acknowledging strategies that were successful, and building a body of information that helps create a clearer vision of what we are trying to do. This includes addressing the issue of sustaining the kinds of skills we've been learning about in this section of the manual on Peer Support and in the next section on WRAP

Evaluating our efforts involves:

1. **Going over a vision, mission, or values statement of the program.**
    The following questions can be used for discussion at the beginning of an evaluation meeting:

    - What is the mission statement for your program?

    - Do your program values and activities, directions and goals fit with your mission statement?

    - If your group or program doesn't have a mission statement, the group may want to work together to develop one. Following is a sample of a mission statement that you could revise for your group:

    Our program is committed to the creation of a safe, supportive, and educational environment for people struggling with a variety of mental health issues. We emphasize understanding, mutual accountability, and respect for diversity. We offer groups and events in which we learn more about ourselves, and how we interact with others. We utilize shared leadership, skill development, team activities and a holistic model of health to make these groups and events a valuable opportunity for growth and strength.

2. **Building a commitment to evaluating interactions in light of the mission and values.** This means assessing activities and interactions using program values as standards. In other words, there should be on-going discussion about day-to-day activities and interactions, in relationship to values. This helps us get away from personal faults and personal criticism. (If you don't know what your program values are, have a discussion about what the mission statement means. Generate a list of values from this discussion).

3. **Discussion about "perception and truth"** (Is there a "right" way?) Go over again what it means to have multiple "truths." Take an example from the week or month. Ask everyone for their perception of the situation. What were people's assumptions? Are there any that are more or less accurate? Why or why not? For example, you might talk about a specific incident from the view of a worker, a member, a guest, a board member.

4. **Discussion about delivering and receiving difficult messages** We might start with a discussion about people's other experiences with critical feedback and evaluation. Recognize that there isn't anyone who absolutely loves getting criticism. We might ask the group if there is anyone that is already feeling particularly sensitive. If so we might ask how they can hear criticism so that it feels helpful. For example, could they clear their defenses so that they can hear it simply as one person's perceptions? Can they sit silently while hearing the feedback? It is then important for them to ask questions so that they can get really clear about others' perceptions.

   Providing criticism also takes skill and awareness. We need to make sure we are not going in with an attitude of feeling self-righteous. It's helpful to start by saying specifically what you noticed without using any judgmental words. For example, "I noticed that you didn't come into work this week, and that you didn't call. Help me understand how that fits with shared responsibility. I feel frustrated because I wasn't sure what else to do other than fill in for you. I ended up feeling resentful without even knowing what was going on for you."

   Or simply asking, "I wonder if you're in a position to hear something potentially difficult?"

5. **Identifying skills that help all people "move through their discomfort."** Sometimes these discussions are going to get more heated. People may find themselves falling into roles that they have used in the past when they were in difficult and even dangerous situations, roles that are not needed in the current situation and inhibit mutual work. How will the whole group take responsibility for sitting with its own discomfort? Who will notice and inform the group when people seem to be sliding into roles? What will people in the group commit to doing when difficult situations arise, things like staying in the room, breathing, being respectful? Things that might help include: taking breaks when needed, passing a talking stick, agreeing to disagree etc.

   Can you think of any others?

   _____

   _____

   _____

   _____

   _____

6. **Helping people become self-reflective and aware.** Find out how individuals are practicing their own values in action. Do they keep an evidence journal? (Evidence journals are notebooks we carry around to note evidence that practicing our values in action is working.) Do they evaluate their day? What's different about their own lives and relationships this week because of values in action?

7. **Evaluating group interactions**. After people have familiarized themselves with the concepts above, they may be prepared to present an interaction or a situation in which a particular value was utilized. This can be something that happened to them or something they observed. Similarly, they could come prepared to offer an interaction or situation that really detracted from Peer Support values, and then describe the results. After each person presents, the group can respond by answering the following questions:

   - What struck them about it?
   - Why did that catch their attention?
   - What personal experience have they had that made them relate to this experience:
   - What has this incident made them think of, that they hadn't been thinking about before they heard about it? (White, 1995)

8. **Finding and articulating an evaluation question to help the program further self evaluate.** Some questions might include:

   - What is the role of someone working at the program, a guest using the respite program, someone who identifies as a member of the program?
   - What happens to mutuality when one person is paid?
   - How is "power" interfering with our ability to "do" help differently?
   - How are we beginning to understand "help" differently?
   - What are the "traps" we fall into?

Program Evaluation

Peer Support programs have been evolving for the last 40 years. While we've helped people decrease their need for traditional services, we've also begun to systematically challenge the dominant assumptions about mental illness and treatment. However, research and evaluation of our programs is often done with methods and hypotheses that don't fit with what we are doing and learning. Research is needed that explores how Peer Support programs create new norms, language, relational roles, and ultimately shift the way we understand mental illness.

There are many approaches to conducting research and evaluation that support the values of Peer Support. Examples include qualitative methods like narrative and participatory action research. These methods give "subjects" the opportunity to also conduct the research.

This may include creating the questions, conducting the interviews, analyzing the data, and deciding how that information will be represented. By exploring different experiences with Peer Support, relationships with mental health systems, and the kinds of things that are "helpful and unhelpful," we can begin to tease apart the unique qualities of Peer Support from other interventions.

One process that we've used in a variety of programs includes the following as described by Cheryl MacNeil (2003):

Phase 1: *Exploration and discovery*–This means asking people about their under-standing of Peer Support, how it's different from mental health services, what it's meant to them in their lives, and what they think the most important qualities are. This can be done through interviews, focus groups, participant observation, journals, and program documents (mission statement, etc.) It is a process that should happen continuously so that the information that's being collected may also show the evolving nature of Peer Support.

Phase 2: *Data collection and analysis*—As information is collected, participants analyze it for significant and repetitive themes that then allow them to identify the dimensions of Peer Support and why they are of value.

Phase 3: *Member checking*— Information is then taken back to the program or group and assessed for accuracy by having the members review it and give feedback.

Phase 4: *Developing our own outcomes and indicators*—New questions will be asked to determine "good outcomes," and then indicators of those outcomes will be identified. Because the mental health system has defined good outcomes as things like treatment compliance, symptom management, etc., we need to make sure Peer Support outcomes like empowerment and recovery are clearly demonstrated. These demonstrations (or performance indicators) may be as simple as numbers of avoided hospitalizations, or in the emergence of themes like unlearning the mental patient role.

Some of the standards and indicators currently being collected by MacNeil are:

Critical Learning **and the re-naming of experiences**— People involved with Peer Support eventually tend to think of themselves, the idea of crisis, their rituals of care, and their relationships with others very differently. Because the trauma-based orientation of the Peer Support culture helps people to better understand how traumas of the past have been viewed through a medical lens, peers begin to redefine who they have become, how they have become, the nature of helping relationships, and what they will need to do to heal. Indicators of this might include people noticing how they've moved out of the "mental patient" identity.

Community—The support received in peer programs and groups gives people a sense of "belonging somewhere." It is a place where you are allowed to be "all" of who you are. Indicators might include increasing numbers of members involved in all aspects of the program/group. They may include a shift in language. Rather than hearing about "clients and consumers," we may begin to hear "people" or "community members."

Flexibility– Peers support each other around individual preferences or needs. Also, peer communities strive to create a range of activities that keep people included. Indicators could come from records of program activities.

Instructive—Peers value each other's expertise and recognize that learning goes both ways. They are both teachers and learners in any given day. If someone comes up with an idea they are encouraged to develop it. When conflict or tension surfaces, it is defined as a learning opportunity. Indicators might include an increase in member-led activities, decrease in conflict, or the extent to which people are able to stay with an uncomfortable process (like conflict).

Mutual Responsibility—It is recognized that every person is equally responsible for making sure that all actions are related to program/group values. Indicators include stories of increased personal and relational responsibility, support going both directions, increased community responsibility for up-keep and success of the program.

Practicing Honesty—It is the expectation that every person involved with Peer Support is honest and respectful. This level of honesty requires that people provide and expect feedback and are able to "handle" it. Success might be indicated by less gossip, more direct communication and less defensiveness.

Setting Limits—Peers have to be clear with themselves and each other about what they can and cannot do and why this is so. This might be identified by less burn-out, people noticing that they're more able to say "no," less gossip and resentment, etc.

Safety —What safety means to each peer and among peers in a Peer Support relationship has to be mutually negotiated. This may involve sitting down together and figuring out what kinds of things allow people to make mistakes, be vulnerable, take risks, etc. Defining safety may also mean that peers develop the right tools and seek information in order to support one another, and that they accept the consequences of making others feel unsafe. Indicators could include movement from the definition of safety as risk management towards safety as creating an environment in which people are supported in trying new things. They may also include an increasing tolerance for working through conflict, people taking responsibility for their actions, and less gossip and blaming. (MacNeil, 2003).

Chapter 11

How Groups Work

As we proceed with taking what we have learned in Peer Support and using it in working together as groups and to develop WRAP, we need to take a look at the different stages of group development: Forming, Storming, and Norming.

Forming

When a group is brand new, people need to know what it's going to be about (information about recovery, general support group, education on specific topic, etc.); what their role is in the group (participant, facilitator, teacher, etc); and what the "rules" are (respectful communication, open to all opinions, no put downs, etc.) The facilitator(s) should have a good idea about the topic or area being explored and should be able to explain it so that people can decide if it's of interest. This is a good time to agree on the purpose of the group while helping everyone understand that members have different levels of anxiety, experience, existing leadership ability and/or lack of confidence. It is also a good time for group members to get to know each other and learn where their beliefs could be similar or different. With this acceptance, the group can get down to work and begin to build a sense of trust.

Starting a group

Groups can take a variety of forms. What kind of activity or format will help people want to attend and be involved in the group? Maybe it would be a trip to a movie, leading to a discussion about courage, empowerment, and recovery. Maybe it will be a skills group like WRAP where people are working on something very specific, both on their own and in the group.

What seem to be some themes in your program? Are people feeling that they've lost their self-confidence or their ability to make good decisions? Do people feel lonely or over-dependent on their case manager for "company"?

> **Exercise:** Each person shares how they think their life will be different if this group is successful. Ask people what their experience has been in other groups and get an idea of what kind of process they will be comfortable with. Generate a set of guidelines that will help everyone do their part to make the group work.
>
> Some guidelines might include:
>
> - Everyone agrees to take responsibility for their own participation.
> - People are on time
> - The group pro-actively decides on the topic
> - There are no "stupid" questions.

Storming

After trust develops and differences are raised, conflict tends to erupt. When this happens, some members may wish to leave the group. Other members become silent. Some people experience irritation with the pace of the group, feeling it is going too fast or too slow.

This is also a stage at which the group wants the facilitator(s) to "fix it." Facilitators in peer groups can help the group work through its own conflict, rather than providing the solution. Further, the role of a Peer Support facilitator is to model Peer Support and to notice (with the group) when it's not happening.

Group members may need to practice working together to get comfortable with conflict and to realize that it is necessary for the growth of the group. Working together, members can come to understand that everybody has a point of view based on his or her experience and history. The facilitator can help group members notice when some difficult dynamic is starting to appear. He or she can then ask the group how they will work through it together. Statements like, "It looks like we are getting off the topic. I wonder how we can get things back on track?" are helpful. It is also very important for the facilitator(s) to model positive risk taking. This might be as simple as saying, "I don't understand." The only way to create trust in a group is to make it safe for all people, including the facilitator, to have their vulnerabilities.

Sometimes attention goes to the facilitator(s) to make decisions. It is important, right from the start, to redirect the attention. As facilitator, don't assume the role of expert. Contribute to the group as a full member. Model that it's okay to say, "I don't know." Trust that the group has the ability to work through difficulties even though it feels uncomfortable.

Norming

Finally, the group tends to get to a level of synergy or working really well together. This means that the group is able to work with differences and access strengths while moving ahead with an agenda. Members take on leadership roles without being bossy. They'll "call themselves" on bad dynamics and they'll have an excitement about what they are learning from each other. It is a time when people build strong connections with each other.

What is most important in understanding group development is that groups may go through all of these processes over and over again. Sometimes this happens when a new person comes to a group, sometimes it simply happens for no reason.

Power in Groups

Have you ever been in a meeting or a group where one person, or maybe a few people, controlled the agenda and took up all the time, or didn't participate until the last minute, and then wouldn't let the meeting adjourn? These are all ways that people can take power in groups and when it happens, the group focus shifts from the original topic and instead revolves around the power struggles. Whether we admit it or not, there are always dynamics of power in groups and in all relationships. Power differences are just that—differences. Some differences that may affect power relationships in groups, but that tend to go unrecognized, are:

- Level of education
- Degree of experience
- Financial difference
- Disability
- Gender difference

These differences are also built into the structure of our culture and society. If we don't recognize these differences, they can lead to difficult behaviors within the group and within all relationships.

It can be useful to model positive power on the individual level. This often comes from a sense of self-confidence and integrity. It is a state in which we are comfortable with our strengths, our vulnerabilities and ourselves. Positive power is also the ability to notice and be respectful of how people's sense of power has been "shot down" (e.g., learning by experience that your opinion makes no difference). Some ways of modeling this kind of positive power include:

- Use your own growth experience as a way of building hope
- Look for the strengths and successes of all members
- Be able to be comfortable enough even when there is conflict
- Believe in all members' abilities
- Being tremendously honest and respectful

Power is often equated with control. People in our lives have taken power when they're afraid, when there's a liability risk, or when we're seen as incapable. Assumptions are made that are not based on fact. It is then that personal power is used to "convince," or even to coerce. An example of this might include someone saying, "I've been in this business for 30 years, you should do it this way."

Some things to notice about group power issues are things like positional power, knowledge power, or personal power. For example: a person's position at their job, more experience or knowledge with a particular topic, or characteristics like charisma, self-confidence or previous experience with leadership positions.

If we find a way for the group to value each member and to recognize that power dynamics exist, we can begin to practice sharing the power. This process will be tremendously important when we as a group confront power on a structural level.

For example did a previously silent member suggest a new topic? Did someone stop when they were talking too much? Did a member, previously prone to giving advice, draw on the strengths and internal resources of another?

Conflict

If we do not attend to conflict in our groups it can lead to resentment, lack of cooperation, lack of energy, people avoiding each other, or in direct attacks. Not only does this make the group less than functional, it will have an impact on the whole program.

Conflict can arise when a member is particularly attached to something. This might mean that they try to convince others that their belief is the "truth." It is important to understand that knowledge and truth are always being created as we share our experiences. An example of this might be a discussion about medications in which group members have an array of different experiences, all of which are true and meaningful for them.

There is no rule that says that a group has to be a place where people sit around in a circle and talk about their problems, or a place to go to "get fixed." We can be really creative in Peer Support; it is just a matter of getting started and sticking with it. **Remember, activities and groups are happening even if only two people attend.**

Section 2

Wellness Recovery Action Planning

Chapter 12

A Description of *WRAP*

I n the last section of this manual we discussed the latest thinking about Peer Support. How is that connected to WRAP? Many of us have been facilitating WRAP groups for years—and doing a great job. And because we have been doing this important work, many of us have made remarkable advances in our journey of recovery. Now we are presented with a new challenge that promises to further enhance the effectiveness of WRAP —using Peer Support methods, skills and strategies in working together to develop Wellness Recovery Action Plans and to support each other as we use these plans to recover and make our lives the way we want them to be.

What is WRAP?

As we said in the first chapter of the book, Peer Support is a new and different way of developing and maintaining relationships, and WRAP is a new and different way of managing life. WRAP is a planning process that involves assessing the self help tools and resources that we have, and then using those tools and resources to develop plans for keeping ourselves well, and for helping ourselves feel better in difficult times. It includes a daily maintenance list, triggers and an action plan, early warning signs and an action plan, when things have gotten much worse and an action plan, crisis planning and post crisis planning.

Before I had a WRAP, I (Mary Ellen) was convinced that I was "manic depressive," that I could never get well, that I had no control over what was happening to me and that I often had no control over my behavior. When I began to feel "too anxious" or "too sad," I called my doctor and got a medication change, or I spent some time in the hospital. Neither of these strategies was ever helpful. As I learned more and more about mental health recovery from people who had some of the same experiences I did, I began to question my label. I was beginning to see that some of the terrible things that had happened to me in my life were causing me to have deep depressions, and out of control behavior. I began to see that I could have more control over what was happening to me and my life, that I could definitely change my behavior and that I could respond to difficult times in different ways when I had sad feelings, suicidal thoughts and severe anxiety.

Now, using WRAP, I do things every day to keep myself well, and if I begin to feel sad, anxious or upset, I have learned that I can live with those uncomfortable feelings without being in any danger. And I can use simple, safe wellness tools to help myself feel better — things like calling or getting together with a peer, reading a good book, making some music, taking a walk or doing some deep breathing.

Anyone can develop a WRAP on their own, using one or several of the resources listed in the appendix of this book. However, many people have found it to be most helpful to develop and use a WRAP while working with a peer who is also developing a WRAP or has already developed a WRAP, or in a Peer Support group. As people work together, they are guided by and learn from the Peer Support strategies described in the beginning chapters of this manual.

In traditional mental health programs, others often developed our treatment and life plans—sometimes without even consulting us. I (Mary Ellen) remember being shown my treatment plan. At the top was a list of goals. But they were not my goals. Someone else had decided what my goals should be. The activities that they described that I was to use to meet these goals were of no interest to me. I even found some of them to be distasteful. Others were trying to take over control of every aspect of my life, including where I would live, who my friends would be, what I would do for work, what I would do with my leisure time, how my "symptoms" would be treated, and what would happen to me if they got worse. This was not at all helpful. It made me feel disempowered and worse than ever.

WRAP is different. WRAP is totally self-determined. There is only one person who can write your WRAP—YOU! (Others can contribute ideas you might never have thought were possible *if you want them to*). You, and only you, decide: If you want to develop a WRAP, how much time it takes you to do it, when you want to do it, what you want and don't want in it, which parts you want to do, who you want, if anyone, to help you with it, how you use it, who you show it to, where you keep it and who, if anyone, knows about it. *If you are developing a WRAP for yourself and someone else tries to interfere with or control your process, explain to them that this is for and by you, and only you can make decisions that are related to your WRAP.*

Why do WRAP and Peer Support work together?

Many of us have begun our healing and recovery after having had years of intense emotional challenges in our lives. We may have had great difficulty being with and/or communicating with others and, as a result, have often been misunderstood. In addition, we may have lived in very isolated, impoverished circumstances at home, in the community or in an institution. After long periods of feeling isolated and being treated badly, we may have forgotten how to relate to others, or perhaps our lives were so traumatic that we never even had the chance to develop healthy relationships. Going to a Peer Support center or group may seem impossible. Peer Support may seem like an almost unattainable goal. And yet many of us report that Peer Support is an important and perhaps essential part of our recovery.

Using WRAP and Peer Support together can help us build strong relationships and community. These can be the first steps in our recovery process. Gradually, through the support and mentoring of others in the groups, we can again become more involved with others, and begin to feel part of the community. We may even choose to connect again with family members and friends who used to be part of our life.

There are other reasons why programs use WRAP and Peer Support together. Some of them may resonate with you. They include:

- Support of individual and group healing as well as relationship and community building
- Similar values, ethics, goals and objectives
- Peer Support centers, and other places where we gather, are ideal places for learning about WRAP and Peer Support, as well as a wealth of other information and opportunities.
- Work together developing Wellness Recovery Action Plans, eliminating hierarchical issues that commonly impede recovery.
- We can support each other as we work on using our plans every day.
- WRAP helps us to make plans for different ways of handling hard times if they occur and Peer Support involves new ways of working through difficult times in our lives.
- We can use WRAP and Peer Support to challenge old ways of thinking and create new ways of thinking
- We may find it easier to work and play together if we are doing what we can to help ourselves feel well while working on mutually responsible relationships.
- WRAP and Peer Support help us to take good care of ourselves and to avoid doing things that sabotage our wellness.

List any other reason why Peer Support and WRAP can be used together.

_____

_____

_____

_____

Expected outcomes from the use of Peer Support and WRAP include:

- Improved quality of life.
- Higher levels of wellness, opportunity and possibility
- Increased use of natural supports
- Personal responsibility and empowerment
- Increased understanding of difficult feelings and behaviors
- Decrease in the incidence of difficult feelings and behaviors
- Decrease in the impact of traumatic life events and stigma caused by difficult feelings and behaviors
- Decrease in the need for costly therapies and health services

The expected long term outcomes of WRAP and Peer Support programs are:

- A shift of focus in mental health care from symptom control to prevention and recovery.

- A significant reduction in the need for costly mental health and emergency services as we effectively take responsibility for our own wellness and stability, manage and reduce difficult feelings and behaviors using a variety of self-help techniques, and effectively reach out for and use the support of a network of peers, family members, friends and health care providers.

- An increased ability to meet life and vocational goals, significant life enhancement, and gains in self-esteem and self-confidence as we become contributing, valued members of the community.

What would you see as other possible outcomes?

_____

_____

_____

General Guidelines for Developing WRAP in Groups

1. Someone or several people may have heard about WRAP and want to work with others developing WRAPs. It can be helpful if several people have been to a series of basic WRAP classes or taken the Mental Health Recovery and WRAP Correspondence Course (see Appendix) where they learned about WRAP. It is even more helpful if one or several people have been to a WRAP training where they learned how to facilitate WRAP groups. These trainings are being held throughout the USA and in other countries. For information on training, ask others at the Peer Support center or refer to the list of contacts in the back of this book.

2. If you want to have a WRAP group and neither you nor any other member has been to a training, you can set up a group and learn WRAP simply by following the process. You can use the information in this manual as a guide, and refer to the resources in the appendix. All you really need to know is the structure of WRAP, the kinds of things that are usually included in each part and, perhaps most important, the values and ethics that will be your guide. The rest of the input comes from the group. The essence of both WRAP and Peer Support is people learning and growing together. The manual _Mental Health Recovery_ including _WRAP Curriculum: A Facilitator's Guide_ (Copeland, revised, 2003, Brattleboro, VT: Peach Press) includes directions for facilitating WRAP groups, a CD-ROM containing the full set of transparencies to guide you through the process, and numerous educational handouts.

3. Enhance the power of WRAP and the WRAP process by using the skills and strategies learned in Peer Support. This may mean discussing issues of power and mutuality, and helping each other move beyond perceived limitations and old roles.

4. Use the resources listed in the appendix as a guide and have them available for easy reference. The transparencies and handouts in *Mental Health Recovery* including *WRAP Curriculum: A Facilitator's Guide* (see Appendix) can guide us through the WRAP process.

5. One or several people in the group who are familiar with WRAP may facilitate the group process. They describe each section of WRAP, share examples and get input from group members. The group could also choose to take turns with facilitation with members being responsible for learning about a section and sharing it with the group. However the group chooses to work together, the group belongs to the group, not to the facilitator, and each group member shares equal responsibility for the work that gets done.

6. Have an easel, plenty of newsprint paper and markers available. After each section of the plan is described, the group shares their ideas. These can be recorded on newsprint, labeling the top of the sheet with the topic, like "Early Warning Signs" or "Wellness Toolbox". Post the list on the wall for easy reference in plan development. Someone in the group could volunteer to input the lists on a computer and print copies for everyone in the group.

7. Most people choose to develop their WRAP in a *three ring binder* with filler paper and a set of five tabs. However, any kind of notebook or paper works. WRAP can also be developed on a *computer* or *tape recorder*. Participants may want to bring binders to the sessions and work on them during the sessions or write notes at the meetings and develop the plan later. In some treatment centers, care providers have insisted on keeping our binders or plans between sessions so we "wouldn't lose them" or so the staff could "check them". This is not OK. These plans are our personal property. If we lose them we either find them or redo them. And no one checks them, or uses them to check up on us.

8. Our own WRAP belongs to each of us and is not to be judged by anyone.

9. WRAP can be created in any order, in any time frame and can be changed at any time. Everything is optional.

10. A person may attend a WRAP session and never write a WRAP. Just being there can be helpful.

11. If all of us who are involved in the group are working on developing or revising a WRAP, we all can give feedback and share information and no one appears to be the "expert."

12. We can encourage each other as we develop our WRAP by saying encouraging things like:

> "That sounds like an idea worth exploring. I wonder if you could think even bigger…" (We might say this if someone appears to be limiting themselves to the things they've been told in the past.) Or, "I once tried this, do you think it might be something you'd like to try?" Or, "Can you think of any other ideas?"

13. Working together as a group, even when we are focused on a common task like developing a WRAP, is not always easy. Using the strategies, methods and skills we continue to learn in Peer Support will assist us. Another thing we can do to ease the process is to develop a list of guidelines together to follow as we work with each other in our WRAP group. The guidelines may be the same as or different from rules you have in your Peer Support center or groups. We share ideas on these guidelines and our suggestions are recorded for posting after the list is complete. Ideas for the list include:

- Avoid criticism (of self or others) and judgments and instead, provide critical reflection (e.g. "I wonder if you might be limiting yourself?")
- Listen respectfully when others are sharing
- Avoid sharing personal information about others outside of the group
- Speak from your own experience
- Treat each other with dignity, compassion and respect

These lists can be added to or changed when the group decides to do so.

14. If one or several people have difficulty following the guidelines, the group can respectfully talk with that person or people, working together using Peer Support methods to come to resolution. Some of the issues that often need attention in groups are:

- People who talk too much
- Someone acting as if they are the expert on everything
- A person who interrupts others
- Someone wanting all the attention paid to their needs
- Joking that interferes with doing the work that others want to do

15. Group members may choose to take time during the sessions to share their life stories or discuss any topics that are mutually agreed upon by the group.

Chapter 13
Getting Started

The first time you get together you may want to discuss the general format of WRAP. Briefly going over each step of the plan enhances understanding. The format is:

- Wellness Toolbox, a list of things a person can do to stay well and to help themselves feel better when they are feeling badly
- Daily Maintenance Plan
- Identifying Triggers & Action Plan
- Identifying Early Warning Signs & Action Plan
- Things Are Breaking Down & Action Plan
- Crisis Planning
- Post Crisis Planning.

Someone could make a list of the parts of the plan and post it on the wall for easy reference, or use the transparency in the *Mental Health Recovery including WRAP Facilitator Manual*.

You may want to discuss the development of the concept of WRAP. It was first developed by a group of people who had been dealing with difficult feelings and behaviors for many years, and who were working on their recovery—people who have had experiences similar to our own. It is often reassuring to know that this is not another "approach" developed, without consulting us, by people who think they know what is best for us.

You may also want to talk about the various ways WRAP can be used in our lives, in addition to helping us stay well and helping us feel better when we are feeling badly. For instance, WRAP can by used as a tool to help insure success when planning life changes like: getting a job, changing jobs, increasing work hours, taking on more responsibilities, getting more education or training, leaving supported housing, moving, beginning or leaving an intimate relationship, working on relationship issues or having a child. It can also be used to address other life issues like: chronic or acute illness, addictions, breaking habits, losing weight, caring for an ill or elderly family member or trying out new interests. The possibilities are almost infinite. You could choose to develop a separate WRAP to deal with each issue you want to address or, you could include these issues all in one WRAP.

Chapter 14

Developing the Wellness Toolbox

The Wellness Toolbox provides the underpinnings for WRAP. This is a list of the various simple, safe self help resources we have discovered that help us stay well, as well as those that help us feel better. These could also be called strengths or assets. This is an empowering first step. Many of us don't see the things we do to help ourselves as strengths or assets. You can discuss some of the common wellness tools that are listed in the various WRAP resources (see Appendix) as well as others we have discovered, even those that you have thought about using but have never tried. Some common Wellness Tools include:

- Peer Support (of course)
- Discussing a difficult issue with the other person involved
- Expressing emotion
- Relaxation exercises
- Getting some rest
- Eating healthy food
- Drinking 8 glasses of water a day
- Going for a walk

Think together about what new tools you might be willing to try (some of these might be: trying something you didn't think you could do; or being really open and honest with a friend (even when it's difficult).

What are the tools you've used successfully? To start the creative juices flowing, we might describe times in our lives when we've felt stuck and then think about what shifted that. This is a great time to reflect back some of the things you've noticed in each other's lives ("Do you remember the time you were stuck and you tried punching pillows instead of hurting yourself?")

You can think about all of your collective resources, helping each other think outside the mental health framework we all have been dependent on. Be creative! What are some things that really make us feel on top of the world? What do we need to do to get more of that? What are the things we need, or can do for each other, when either one of us starts slipping?

Working together, groups often come up with long lists of wellness tools. I (Mary Ellen) have learned that when I am feeling badly or trying to keep myself well, there is always a simple, safe wellness tool I can use. I used to reach for a medication or call a crisis line, but I don't have to do that anymore. One of the wellness tools I use most is Peer Support. I call a friend, we talk about what I am experiencing and we share ideas on what might help. Usually that is all I need to feel better.

Some of us have actually developed a physical wellness toolbox: a basket, box, drawer or shelf where we keep wellness tools or reminders of wellness tools, things like a poetry book, a box of watercolors, massage lotion, a relaxation tape, a journal, etc. Another idea is hanging the list of wellness tools on the refrigerator for quick and easy reference.

Occasionally, someone finds the Wellness Toolbox so helpful and the idea that they can use these simple, safe tools to help themselves, they don't choose to go any further with the plan at this time. Others of us may just want to listen to the discussion and not write anything down.

When we talk in our groups about alcohol, substance use, or self-injury, people tend to get very uncomfortable. For some of us, however, these are tools we've developed to survive very difficult situations. Although these activities are often judged negatively and severely, if we think about context again, they may make perfect sense. The issue becomes more complex when people still cite and use them as wellness strategies.

If we refer back to the values and ethics of WRAP and peer support, one of the main values is non-judgment. It is not useful or even respectful to judge someone based on what they do to cope. But we must also consider the value of shared responsibility; perhaps we can begin to talk about what's going to work both for individuals and for the group. For example, would it ever be OK for people to talk about the need/want to harm themselves, in order to relieve the pressure of keeping it secret? Would it be OK if people were working towards abstinence, but taking small steps, like having one less beer a day for a while and then reducing it more?

In the past this has not been an option. It has not been OK to say we feel like hurting ourselves, for fear we'd end up hospitalized or in seclusion and restraints. Or that we were going to continue to drink, but do it less and less. This has only served to set us way back, adding more on to the original trauma.

Recovery is for most of us a gradual process. Over time we use wellness tools, coping strategies and other activities to help us get through difficult times. As we begin to recover, the strategies we use may be very different from those we would use later on. We don't need to expect ourselves, nor should others expect us to make major changes all at once. For instance, it is unreasonable to expect a person to stop cutting, begin therapy and get in the habit of eating three healthy meals a day all at the same time. These changes happen gradually and we need to decide for ourselves if we will make these changes, when we will make these changes and how we will make them. What we can do with each other is to be honest, to support each other in ways that work for us and enhance the relationship, and to remind each other that we're all capable of recovery (even when one of us is not so sure).

Most of us choose to change our WRAP over time as we learn more about ourselves, while building strong relationships. We learn about new tools and strategies from each other and we get better and better at negotiating with each other in advance. For instance, as we begin our recovery, self-harm may still be a coping strategy that we use to get through those times when the emotional pain is so intense. As we work on our recovery, we may find that we are able to call each other and talk about the urge without actually acting on it. Gradually we may harm ourselves less and less as we use our WRAP to help ourselves feel better and to prevent more difficult times. We may find other wellness tools, like expressing our emotions, going for a run, or doing some hard work, gradually reduce our feelings of needing to hurt ourselves. We may also find that we are spending more time with people who are loving and supportive and staying away from people who treat us badly, and that we have made changes in our lives, like getting our own living space, furthering our education, getting a job or doing volunteer work, that increase our overall sense of well being.

When you first develop your WRAP, letting go of an addiction to alcohol may not even be a goal you choose to work on. You may decide that in order to begin your recovery, you need to brush your teeth, comb your hair and change your shirt every day. At some later time you may choose to work on stopping drinking. That is up to you.

Just like anyone else, we lose the right to make choices about the things we do, and the coping strategies that we use, when they have a negative affect on the lives of others. For instance, it's not OK to abuse a child or stalk someone. If we do things that violate others' rights or put others in danger, then we should expect to be prosecuted just like anyone else. Having a psychiatric diagnosis, or having extreme feelings, is not an excuse for hurting others or breaking the law.

The structure and support of the WRAP group, the values and ethics of Peer Support, the participant guidelines and the feelings of mutuality that exist in these groups, make it possible for people to talk openly about things that they have never talked about anywhere else and that they may never have admitted to anyone. For instance, this may be the first place a person can talk without fear about self-harm, or about hiding liquor or stockpiling drugs. Many people report that sharing these experiences with others who are supportive takes away the power of these feelings and actions and allows the person to make changes and move forward with their recovery. Good facilitators and supportive peers recognize and encourage these important conversations. Group members who do not want to be part of these conversations can choose to leave the group for that time.

Chapter 15
The Daily Maintenance Plan

The next step in the WRAP process is developing a Daily Maintenance Plan. It includes three parts:

- What I'm like when I'm well,
- A list of things I need to do every day to stay well,
- A list of things I might need to do to stay well.

If you are using a binder, you can write Daily Maintenance List on the first tab and insert it into the binder followed by several sheets of filler paper.

The first part is **what I'm like when I'm well**. This serves as a reference point. If you have been feeling badly for a long time, you may not remember what feeling well is. For example, I would describe myself as cheerful, loving, outgoing, reflective, risk taking and over achieving. When I have been "down in the dumps" for a week or two, it helps me to refer to this list. Some of us can't recall ever feeling well. In that case, you may want to write what you would like to feel like. A simple list will suffice. Talking with each other about this or discussing it in the group is often fun and thought provoking. It is especially interesting and validating when we share things about ourselves that others have labeled "symptoms," like introverted, talkative, boisterous and argumentative. This exercise can also give validation, self-acceptance and acceptance of others, and normalize our experiences.

On the next page, you list those **things you feel you need to do every day to stay as well as possible**. I know if I did the things on my **Daily Maintenance List** every day, I would feel a lot better. I have kept my list short enough so on most days I can do it. I have a personal rule that I will not "give myself a hard time" if I don't do everything on the list. The following sample plan is what I try to do for myself every day.

- Eat three healthy meals and three healthy snacks
- Drink at least six 8-ounce glasses of water
- Exercise for at least half an hour
- Get half an hour exposure to outdoor light
- 20 minutes of relaxation or meditation
- Write in my journal for at least 15 minutes
- Spend half an hour enjoying a fun, affirming or creative activity

Discussions about the Daily Maintenance List might focus on times in our lives when we felt really good, what that was like and reasons why we felt really good. For instance, if a person said they felt really good when they spent time with their pets, they might want to include that on their daily list.

Some of us have spent years of our lives in institutions or in group homes where we had little or no control over our lives. We may still be living in situations like that. WRAP is a good place to start taking back control of our lives and the Daily Maintenance List is a good place to begin. We can start looking at small things that we can do each day, like making our own bed in the morning, deciding what we want and don't want to eat and which groups we want to attend, going for a longer walk, spending extra time talking to people we like, cutting back on cigarettes or coffee, or simply challenging ourselves to try something brand new. Talking with our peers can help us to figure this out. Our list can be very short to start with. As doing the things on our daily maintenance list becomes easier, we can add things to the list. We may decide to take actions that give us back more and more control over our lives, including moving out of supervised situations and living on our own or with a family member or peer.

Some of us may have troubling feelings and experiences that are so intrusive that developing a Daily Maintenance List can seem impossible. For instance, if we are constantly hearing voices and have extreme anxiety and fear, it may be difficult to think of things we can do to keep ourselves well. This is another time when the list can be very short. For instance, a list might be one thing—I will smile at one person each day or I will look one person in the eye. It may even be as simple as I'll brush my teeth without being reminded, eat a piece of fruit or walk around the building outside. These can be significant first steps toward recovery. Having peers to talk to as we are developing these lists and making these changes in our lives affirms us in this life changing process.

The next part of this section is a list of things we don't always need to do, but that we might need or want to do sometimes. Some of these things, like paying bills, will create extra stress in our lives if we don't do them. As with each preceding section, we work together as individuals or groups, discussing the section and sharing ideas, writing down those ideas that resonate with us in our own plans. Some ideas for this list include:

- Spend time with a good friend or a Peer Supporter
- Spend extra time with my partner
- Be in touch with my family
- Spend time with children or pets
- Buy groceries
- Pay bills
- Get more sleep
- Have some personal time
- Plan something fun for the weekend
- Plan a vacation
- Go for a long walk
- Go to a support group

Chapter 16

Triggers, Early Warning Signs & When Things are Breaking Down

We use the same process we used in developing the Daily Maintenance List as we work our way through the next three sections of WRAP—Triggers, Early Warning Signs and When Things are Breaking Down, inserting a tab for each section if we are using a binder, describing and discussing the section, and getting ideas from each other as we proceed. Each of these sections includes a listing of difficulties or uncomfortable feelings and responses or actions we could take in these situations.

Triggers

The Triggers section has been important to me. In the past, when I was in my "mental illness" persona, if something bad happened to me or was upsetting (a trigger), I either got very upset, went into a panic, got confused, lashed out at someone or something, or engaged in some other behavior that was both self defeating and isolating. Sometimes I didn't even know what the trigger was. The situation often escalated to the point that someone would suggest I needed more medication, tried to control me in some way, or ostracized me. This made me feel worse and worse. Often the end result of this was what I then referred to as a "crisis," which I thought, and others confirmed, was a result of my "mental illness".

Now all of that has changed. I recognize my triggers: people treating me badly, being overtired, feeling left out, traumatic news stories. Using my Wellness Toolbox, I have developed a list of actions I can use that will help me get through this difficult time without resorting to the old behaviors that are remnants of a difficult childhood and several abusive adult relationships. These actions may help me to feel better or resolve the situation, and may also encourage interaction and support from others. Now when I am triggered, if another person is involved, I can choose from any number of options depending on the circumstances. These might include discussing the situation with the other person, calling a peer and discussing it with her or him, writing about it in a journal, choosing to forget about it by immersing myself in a good book or playing my drums, going to my room to pound the pillows and cry, taking a few deep breaths, or having a rambunctious romp with my dog. If it is a more serious trigger, like a serious illness, I might call a supporter to discuss a plan for dealing with the situation over time.

In my WRAP I have listed some of my triggers as:

- Anniversary dates of losses or trauma
- Traumatic news events
- Being overly tired

- Family friction
- Spending too much time alone
- Being judged, criticized, teased or put down
- Financial problems
- Physical illness
- Sexual harassment
- Feeling unsafe
- Feeling left out
- Coming into contact with things that remind me of abandonment or deprivation
- Intimacy
- Excessive stress
- Extreme guilt
- Substance abuse

Some of the tools I have listed in my Action Plan for responding to Triggers include:

- Planning ahead for difficult times
- Discussing the situation with a peer
- Avoiding reading the newspaper and watching the news on television
- Avoiding people who treat me badly
- Doing something I really enjoy
- Playing the piano
- Doing a deep breathing exercise

For some people, the word "trigger" means things are out of control and there is nothing they can do about it. Sometimes we also may accuse others of triggering us (this is blaming and is also inaccurate). A trigger can become an excuse and put us back in that old victim role. We stay out of that role when we respond in ways that support wellness, recovery and relationships with others. For example, a woman was in a restaurant having lunch with a group of friends. One of the friends made a comment that was very embarrassing to her. She yelled at the other woman, threw a glass of water in her face and stormed out of the restaurant. Afterward she felt embarrassed and humiliated by her own actions. She also noticed that friends stopped including her in invitations. In considering this event and discussing it with her peers, she realized there were other ways she could have handled the situation. She could have told the woman that she was embarrassed and asked her not to do it again. She could have asked the woman to go outside with her to discuss the situation. She could have asked another friend to go outside and talk with her to do a reality check and figure out how to handle it. She could have taken a time out and gone to the rest room to think about it. She could have ignored it until later and spoken with the women who embarrassed her afterward. There were lots of options. When we get together to work on WRAP, we may want to share some situations we have experienced and discuss possible solutions—new ways of responding to troubling situations.

Early Warning Signs

The next section is Early Warning Signs. These are subtle signs that things are not quite right. When we experience early warning signs, we may be unclear about why we feel the way we do, but we notice that we feel different. Or, sometimes, early warning signs are so subtle we hardly notice them at all. Discussing early warning signs with peers can increase our awareness of these signs and help us recognize those that we may not have thought of as signs. Some examples of early warning signs are:

- Anxiety or nervousness
- Forgetfulness
- Lack of motivation
- Feeling slowed down or speeded up
- Avoiding doing things on my Daily Maintenance List
- Avoiding others or isolating
- Beginning irrational thought patterns
- Increased irritability or negativity
- Increase in smoking
- Not keeping appointments
- Spending money impulsively
- Feelings of discouragement or hopelessness
- Substance abuse
- Failing to buckle my seat belt
- Not answering the phone
- Overeating or under-eating

I used to ignore early warning signs. I just kept "pushing through" and hoping they would go away. Usually the opposite happened. I felt worse and worse and worse. Now when I notice early warning signs, I take action. And when I do, the early warning signs usually go away and I feel fine again. Sometimes it's hard to take action, but I have learned that my best strategy is to persist. The other people in my life appreciate my efforts almost as much as I do.

I also used to think of early warning signs as something that were out of my control- making me worry about what others might see as normal difficult feelings. Because I've worked hard to identify those signs, I can make choices about how I want to handle them. Now I'm not afraid of my own feelings and others aren't afraid for me.

Discussing action plans with peers when we have early warning signs is very useful in ensuring a healthy response. Some ideas of things we could do in response to early warning signs include:

- Talk to a peer (this appears on all of my lists and is the number one best wellness tool I have)
- Do the things on my Daily Maintenance List whether I feel like it or not
- Do at least three 10-minute relaxation exercises each day
- Write in my journal for at least 15 minutes each day
- Spend at least 1 hour involved in an activity I enjoy
- Ask others to take over my household responsibilities for a day
- Go to a support group meeting if there is one

Each part of the plan is a bit more challenging than the last. We can reward ourselves after we complete each section. Make some popcorn. Play a game. Watch a movie. Definitely take plenty of breaks.

When Things are Breaking Down

The next section of the plan is "When Things are Breaking Down". If we have reached this point, we feel really awful, or perhaps we feel wonderful but our peers are telling us that our behavior is unusual or troubling. This is an important time. We can make a decision to do something about it, and that may be hard, or we can just allow the troubling feelings and behaviors to take control. The choice is up to us.

We may want to begin working on this section by discussing with our peers times when things were breaking down in the past, looking at what happened just before we felt that way. We might remember that we lost our job, had a hassle with social security or had a troubling visit with family members. Perhaps we were very over tired or had been eating a lot of junk food. This can help us in identifying the signs that things are breaking down and choosing actions we can take to help us feel better.

We can work with our peers and make a list of signs that will show us we need to take action and decide the actions that we feel would be most helpful. We can also discuss those signs that are indicators that things have gotten much worse and include them in the "When Things are Breaking Down" section of our WRAP. By this time the signs are usually obvious, if not to others, at least we are aware of them. They might include things like:

- Feeling very oversensitive and fragile
- Irrational responses to events and the actions of others

- Feeling very needy
- Unable to sleep for .... (how long?)
- Sleeping all the time
- Avoiding eating
- Wanting to be totally alone
- Racing thoughts
- Risk taking behaviors, e.g. driving too fast
- Thoughts of self-harm
- Being obsessed with negative thoughts
- Inability to slow down
- Bizarre behaviors
- Disassociation (blacking out, spacing out, losing time)
- Seeing things that aren't there
- Taking out anger on others
- Chain smoking
- Spending excessive amounts of money (say how much that means for you)
- Food abuse
- NOT feeling
- Suicidal thoughts
- Paranoia

In the past, many of us would have called a crisis line, asked for additional meds or to be admitted to a hospital when we had these feelings or behaviors. Now we know that is not necessary and is often not in our best interest. Instead we can use our wellness tools and the action plan we have developed for dealing with difficult times.

Again, working together, we develop a plan of what we can do to help ourselves if things are breaking down. The plan now needs to be very directive with fewer choices and clear instructions. A few years ago I developed a plan to use at this time. I showed it to my spouse. My plan included not working for three days. He wondered if I could really do it. So I decided to try. I did a "dry run" of my "When Things are Breaking Down" action plan. And he was right. The first time I couldn't do it. But I still thought it was a good plan. So I tried it again and the second time I was successful.

After identifying feelings and behaviors, we can discuss our plans with each other, report our successes and failures and refine them to improve their effectiveness. We may get some ideas from the following list:

- Call and talk as long as I need to a Peer Supporter

- Arrange for someone to stay with me around the clock until I feel better
- Make sure I am doing everything on my Daily Maintenance List
- Arrange for at least three days off from any responsibilities
- Have at least two peer counseling sessions daily
- Do three deep breathing relaxation exercises daily
- Write in my journal for half an hour
- Spend at least one hour exercising
- Spend at least two hours doing something I really enjoy

One thing we can think about at this time is discomfort. We may have been led to believe that it is not OK to feel uncomfortable. We were taught that if you don't feel fine, you need to take a pill, reach out to a health care provider, or perhaps be admitted to a health care facility for treatment. In developing our plans we may want to think about just being with our discomfort, examining it, responding to it in some way like crying, fussing, whining (to ourselves or a willing listener) or ignoring it. If we wait it out, it may just go away. We could discuss in our group the times when we stayed with our discomfort and what happened. Perhaps we can use "staying with our discomfort" as a wellness tool and include it in our action plans

Completing the Wellness Toolbox and the first four sections of WRAP is a major achievement. By this time we may be seeing ourselves in new ways and feeling we have more power and control over our own lives.

Chapter 17
Crisis & Post Crisis Planning

A crisis plan is the same as, or similar to, an advanced directive. It is a document that is supposed to tell others what we want them to do to take care of us when we can't take care of ourselves. Many mental health systems are mandating that every person who uses their services must have a crisis plan or advanced directive in their file. However, mandated plans, often developed by someone else on our behalf, rarely work. As with the rest of WRAP, we need to develop these plans for ourselves when we feel ready to do so. **It can be kept in an agency file only if we want it to be there.**

If we develop these crisis plans ourselves and if the plan is followed, it keeps us in control, even when it may feel like things are out of control. Others will be doing things with us and for us that are truly helpful, rather than things they **think** might be helpful or **should** be done. In the past, when things were done to us that others thought would be helpful or that were for the convenience of an institution, we generally felt worse. Having our own crisis plan should prevent things like coercion, restraint, isolation and forced medication from happening. **In writing our plans we must be very clear about what we do and don't want to have happen to us.** All of this is good material for discussions with peers.

In our crisis plan we need to be very clear about when we want others to step in and what we want them to do. In addition, we need to be very clear about what we don't want them to do and what we can do for ourselves. Remember, the only time we really can't help ourselves is if we are unconscious. Otherwise we still have our minds and/or our bodies, as well as our peers, as resources we can use to help ourselves.

While other parts of WRAP are only for the use of the person who is developing it, the intent of the Crisis Plan is that it will be given to others when it is completed so they will know how to be of assistance to us when needed. It needs to be written so others can easily understand what we mean. It is up to us to decide whom we want to give it to—whom we want to assist us and whom we don't want to assist us. In writing the plan, we need to describe situations, circumstances and actions in ways that others can clearly understand. When you have completed it, you may want to ask the people you list as supporters to read it over and discuss it with you so they understand your intentions.

Most of us find that developing the crisis plan is the hardest part of WRAP, and that it usually takes more time to develop than all of the other sections of WRAP combined. We may choose to work on it only when we are with a peer or in a group or we may want to complete it on our own.

There is a form for the crisis plan in the Appendix. However, we have the option of developing a new form or changing the one that is provided to better meet our specific needs.

The first section of the crisis plan is the same as part one of the Daily Maintenance section of WRAP—it describes **what we are like when we are well.** Most of us like to have a description of what we are like when we are well at the beginning of the plan in case someone we have never met at an agency or care facility is using the plan. If they don't know what we are like when we are well, they might make some invalid assumptions, assuming some of our behaviors are "symptoms" rather than just part of how we usually are. For instance, we might be very quiet. Someone might assume it is because we are depressed or withdrawn. To avoid that situation, we can easily copy the section "What I'm like when I'm are well" from the beginning of our WRAP. We can also choose to describe ourselves in different ways for the crisis plan. We could do it in a list form, sentences or even write several paragraphs that we feel reflect who we are.

The next section of the plan is a listing of **behaviors or signs** that others would notice that would let them know when we need assistance and support. This takes a lot of thought. Discussions with peers can help us decide what we want to put in this section. We can discuss other difficult times we have had, and when we wish others had been there to assist and support us. This discussion often leads us to rethink our definition of a crisis or what a crisis really is for us. For instance, Mary Ellen wrote the following about her experience:

> I used to think I was in a crisis when I was feeling very agitated and anxious, and when I was crying a lot. Then I realized, there are lots of things I can do to help myself at that time, and it isn't really a crisis at all. I can certainly call a peer or go to the peer center. I can do some of my relaxation techniques. I can take a long walk. I began to think that the only time I am really in a crisis and need others to take over for me is if I am comatose, or so lethargic I literally can't move to feed myself, or if I am hurting myself or threatening to hurt others. Everything that used to be on my old list, things like pacing, counting things over and over and not getting out of bed are things I can manage in the "when things are breaking down" section, using my action plan and Peer Support.

The next section of the crisis plan is a listing of **supporters** who we would want to assist us if we were having a very difficult time. Most of us prefer to have as many peers, family members and friends on the list as possible, limiting the use of care providers, who may not be available or who may be dealing with agency boundary issues. This list can include contact information such as phone numbers and E-mail so supporters can be in touch with each other. Preferences about supporters who can meet specific needs can also be listed. Most of us find that at least five supporters is a good number. It assures that someone will be available. Most of us have fewer than that to start, but work on building our list over time. As peers we can discuss the kinds of attributes we want our supporters to have as well as good and bad experiences with supporters in difficult times.

Most people also want to include a list of people they do not want involved if they are having a difficult time. It could be a doctor, family member or care provider. This may be someone who has treated us badly in the past. This is not a time to worry about hurting someone's feelings by not including them. This is about each of us and what we need.

The next section is straightforward. It is a listing of **medications / supplements / health care preparations** we are using, when we use them and why we are using them. It can also include contact information for our physician and pharmacist, as well as insurance information. This section includes a list of medications that are acceptable to us if medications are needed, as well as those that must be avoided. Often peers will want to discuss the benefits and liabilities of taking medications or of certain medications. This discussion can get in the way of other more helpful conversations. It also helps if peers agree not to try and directly influence people's choices around medications. An activity might be gathering lots of books on medications, having access to the internet, and spending some time together studying the pros and cons of medications and learning the specifics of certain medications.

In the next section, **Treatments and Complementary Therapies,** we list acceptable and unacceptable treatments and complementary therapies like acupuncture and massage. Electroshock therapy can be an issue here. As we are developing our list of treatment options, we may want to study the pros and cons of electroshock and other possible options.

The next section of the plan, **Home Care / Community Care / Respite Center,** is very important. In these days of budget cuts, limited access to services and brief hospital stays, a person can benefit by having a comprehensive plan that would allow them to stay at home and/or part time in a facility in the community when they are having difficulties. Hopefully there is a peer run respite center available in your area. Many of us would feel better much more quickly if we're at home in our familiar surroundings with our own things and people who know us close by. Following is an example of a plan:

I don't like to go to the hospital because I can lose some of my rights when I am there. I am expected to attend groups and activities that don't meet my needs, I have to follow their schedule which can be upsetting, and I don't like the food. On the other hand, if it were a really good facility, I would appreciate a "time out". Given that such a facility does not exist, I have developed a comprehensive plan that would allow me to stay at home or in the community in almost all circumstances.

Topics for discussion among peers might include the pros and cons of hospitalization, community options, respite facilities and families' abilities to provide intensive care.

Plans that others have developed have included a mix of things like: going to a respite center, having family members and friends stay with you for certain periods of time, spending part of the day in a treatment center and having family members or peers provide support for the rest of the day. Developing this part of the plan takes careful consideration and extra time.

In the next section we list our choices of **hospital or treatment facilities** should they become necessary. Many of us have found that, using WRAP, we have fewer or no hospitalizations. A group discussion of the ideal treatment facility can be fun and thought provoking. For instance, I believe every treatment center should have hot tubs or Jacuzzis that are available whenever people want to use them. Some of us have felt so strongly about the needs for change in these facilities that we have made it the focus of our advocacy work.

A listing of hospitals and treatment facilities to be avoided might also be included.

The next section of the plan is **Help from others**. It deserves extra attention and discussion. Many of us have never taken the time or been encouraged to think about what others can do for us that would be helpful in difficult times. Our supporters have usually done what they felt was best without asking us for input. This may have included the use of coercion, restraint, isolation and forced medication—tactics that can make us feel much, much worse, at a time when we desperately want to feel better. Peers' discussions around this issue will help expand our thinking about what is possible at this time. Some of the things people have written in their plans include:

- Ask me what happened
- Ask me what I want and need
- Hold me
- Don't touch me
- Listen to me without giving me any advice
- Let me express my emotions
- Let me do what I need to do
- Make me macaroni and cheese
- Get me funny videos to watch
- Cook me a healthy meal
- Listen closely to what I say

In addition it could include a list of **things we need to have done for us** like:

- Buy some groceries
- Call my boss and tell him I have a cold
- Pay the rent
- Feed the pets
- Care for the children (if a person has children, it is important that they have a carefully designed alternative plan that provides for care of the children)

This section can also include a **list of things people might do that would not be helpful and would make us feel worse**, like:

- Correcting me
- Giving me advice
- Nagging
- Scolding
- Blaming or shaming me

- Teasing me
- Trying to divert me with chatter
- Inviting lots of my friends to come over
- Playing certain kinds of music
- Describing bad times others have had
- Threats or abuse
- Restraint

In the next section of the plan, **Inactivating the Plan,** we list indicators that let others know when they no longer need to follow the plan—that we no longer need intensive support. The list might include things like: when I am cooking for myself and eating three healthy meals each day, when I am not afraid to go outside, when I am no longer pacing, or when I return to dressing as I usually do. Again, a discussion of this topic can help us develop ideas.

These plans are a guide for the people who we choose to assist us. In some places they are legally binding, but in many they are not. However, good supporters are delighted to get this kind of information and do the best they can to do as we wish. Even when they are legal, they may not be followed. However, most of us still feel they give us the best chance of getting the care we need and deserve.

In places where the plans are legal, find out whose signatures you need to have the plan legally recognized. Even where it is not legal, it may be of benefit to get the plan signed by an attorney and several witnesses. This increases the likelihood that others will take it seriously and follow your directions.

When this plan is completed, we can distribute copies to our supporters. Some of us have held gatherings of our supporters, or met with them individually, to talk about the plan and its implementation. Supporters may want to give input on parts of the plan they feel would work well, possible problem areas and suggestions for revisions.

Post Crisis Plan

The last section of WRAP is the **Post Crisis Plan**. The Post Crisis Plan was developed several years after the original WRAP. People saw the need for thinking about and planning for that time when we are getting over a hard time and working toward feeling well. This part of the plan differs from other parts of the plan because while some sections can be addressed or partially addressed in advance, many parts of the post crisis plan need to be addressed as we are beginning to feel better. The responses will be dependent on our situation at that time.

In working with the group on this section of the plan, simply describe each part of the plan as listed below, and ask the group for ideas on what might be included in that section. The

Post Crisis Plan form consists of questions we can ask ourselves, either before the hard time (the one we hope will never happen), or when we are beginning to feel better. Each of them is a good topic for group discussion. As with the rest of WRAP, we skip over any questions that aren't meaningful to us or that, for whatever reason, we don't feel like addressing. The actual Post Crisis Plan form is in the Appendix. The questions to be completed include:

- I will know that I am "out of the crisis" and ready to use this post crisis plan when I am able to:

- How I would like to feel when I have recovered from this crisis:

- People I want to support me as I heal:

- Will I feel safe and be safe at home? ___y ___n
  If your answer is no, you may want to respond to the following question:

- What will I do to ensure that I will feel and be safe at home?

- I would like to stay (where) _____ for (how long) _____ before I go home.

- I would like _____ or _____ to take me home.

- I would like _____ or _____ to stay with me.

- When I get home I would like to _____ or _____.

- If the following things are in place, it would ease my return:

- Things I must take care of as soon as I get home:

- Things I can ask someone else to do for me:

- Things that can wait until I feel better:

- Things I need to do for myself every day while I am recovering from crisis:

- Things I might need to do every day while I am recovering from this crisis:

- Things and people I need to avoid while I am recovering from this crisis:

- Signs that I may be beginning to feel worse—anxiety, excessive worry, overeating, sleep disturbances:

- Wellness tools I will use if I am starting to feel worse:

- What do I need to do to prevent further repercussions from this crisis—and when I will do these things?

- People I need to thank:

- People I need to apologize to:

- People with whom I need to make amends:

- Medical, legal, or financial issues that need to be resolved:

- Things I need to do to prevent further loss—like canceling credit cards, getting official leave from work if it was abandoned, cutting ties with destructive friends

- Signs that this post crisis phase is over and I can return to using my Daily Maintenance Plan as my guide to things to do for myself every day:
- Changes in the first four sections of my Wellness Recovery Action Plan that might help prevent such a crisis in the future:
- Changes in my crisis plan that might ease my recovery:
- Changes I want to make in my lifestyle or life goals:
- What did I learn from this crisis?
- Are there changes I want or need to make in my life as a result of what I have learned?
- If so, when and how will I make these changes?

The Post Crisis Plan can also include a **Timetable for Resuming Responsibilities** that others may have had to take over or that did not get done while we were having a hard time. Things like child care, pet care, your job, cooking and household chores. The following sample is a format that could be used for this part of the plan:

SAMPLE: Responsibility: getting back to work

While I am resuming this responsibility, I need (who) *my spouse* to *drive me to work so I don't have to take the bus.*

Plan for Resuming Responsibilities

- In three days go back to work for 2 hours a day for five days
- For one week go to work half time
- For one week work 3/4 time
- Resume full work schedule

Responsibility _____ Who has been doing this while I was in crisis _____

While I am resuming this responsibility, I need (who) _____

to _____

Plan for resuming

_____

_____

_____

_____

_____

Chapter 18

Using WRAP &
WRAP Follow up

At this time some of us will have completed our WRAP. Others will have completed some parts of the plan. Others may have gotten off to a good start. Still others may not have even begun to develop a plan. In any case, participants will have gotten what they needed to get from working through this process or part of this process. Some may have needed to write out the complete plan. Others may have benefited from understanding that they have resources available that they can use to help themselves feel better. For many it may be their first exposure to the concepts of personal responsibility and self-determination.

Using WRAP

After we have finished developing our WRAP, we may want to spend time every day reviewing our work and taking action when we decide it is needed. Morning, either before or after breakfast, is often a good time to review the book. As we become more familiar with it, the review process will take less time and we will know how to respond to certain situations without even referring to the book.

Evaluating a WRAP Group

Evaluating the WRAP group gives vital information that informs future work. We can do this using the Peer Support evaluation methods described in Chapter 10, Evaluating Our Efforts.

Follow up WRAP Support Groups

At the end of the WRAP class, we have often formed significant bonds with each other. We may choose to keep meeting on a regular basis, weekly, every other week, or monthly, to share successes and challenges, to give each other feedback and to provide mutual support. The group can be very informal. A facilitator is not necessary. Members of the group may decide that each person gets a set period of time to talk—like 10 minutes—to assure that everyone in the group gets time to share. Groups are often held at the Peer Support center and may be part of other Peer Support activities. In addition, lots of support concerning WRAP happens informally as people gather to chat and share their experiences.

Chapter 19
Developing a WRAP for Your Group or Program

We have talked at length about using WRAP to enhance individual wellness. WRAP can also be used to deepen relationships, hold groups accountable to their task, and to help whole programs work towards their mission and vision. Peer programs may find this a particularly helpful tool as they are attempting to put their values into day-to-day practice and resolve conflicts. WRAP for your group or program is developed by the members. It could be all the members, or a group that is representing all of the group. It is a group activity that is guided by Peer Support methods and values. You could have a separate meeting to develop each part of the plan or you could do the whole plan in one or several meetings.

You may want to use the same method for developing WRAP for your program that is used when individuals work together in groups to develop their WRAP. One person may take the role of facilitator, several people may share that role, or members of the group take turns facilitating. The facilitator describes the section of the plan that is being addressed. The group may want to discuss it to assure common understanding. Then, using a flip chart for recording responses, participants share their suggestions.

However, in developing the group WRAP, if anyone disagrees with a suggestion, agreement with others must be reached before a suggestion becomes part of the plan. In developing a personal WRAP, the individual is the only person who determines what goes in the plan.

When the plan is complete, someone could enter it into a computer and make copies for group members so everyone has it available for easy reference.

Developing a Vision Statement

The first step in developing a WRAP for your group or organization may be to develop a vision statement. A vision statement is different from the mission statement. A vision statement is the hope and dreams of your program or group. This statement can help programs stay on the edge of learning. In other words, the vision is the living potential of the program. Maybe your long-term vision is that Peer Support will change the way mental illness is understood, influence treatment, offer people a fully viable alternative to traditional services, and provide a resource that will enhance meaningful community integration. This vision is what keeps us trying, keeps us moving ahead, and gives us hope as we sometimes struggle.

When I (Shery) first got involved with a Peer Support program, my vision was to create a hospital alternative. Up until that point I'd had many hospitalizations that left me feeling shameful, isolated, broke and broken. I had also had some experience with healing relationships that were mutual and non-judgmental. Those healing relationships convinced that with the right training, and the right thinking, we could create a program that would offer people a chance to work through their most difficult times with the support and compassion of friends. Not just friends in a crisis, but also long term friends who would help us learn and grow. Two years after we opened the peer program, we were funded to open New Hampshire's first peer run crisis respite program. That program has now kept literally hundreds of people from being hospitalized when they are having a difficult time.

If we start with the vision rather than the mission of our organizations, we can use WRAP to move beyond maintenance and strive to achieve things we may not even know we are capable of.

Write a vision statement (a statement of hopes and dreams) with members of your group for your group or program.

_____

_____

_____

_____

Wellness Toolbox for Programs

The next step in developing a WRAP for your group or program is to develop a Wellness Toolbox, a list of things your group can do assure that it works toward its vision. This is a group process. Everyone in the group gets together and develops this list. These tools will be used to develop the rest of the Wellness Recovery Action Plan for your group or program.

The wellness toolbox for your group might include:

- Weekly evaluation and reflection
- Strategic planning
- People maintaining responsibility
- Communicating directly
- Practicing Peer Support values
- Working through conflict
- Holding a special meeting
- Having a retreat day
- Doing a fun activity together
- Having a celebration
- Delegating tasks

- Problem solving activities
- Working with a mediator
- Changing your meeting space
- Giving one-on-one support
- Brainstorming
- Collaborating with others
- Consultation with an expert
- Having a special presentation

The members of your group will think of many other ideas. What are some of your group's wellness tools?

- _____
- _____
- _____
- _____
- _____
- _____

Describe the Group When Things are Going Well

Next in our WRAP we think about what our program/group looks, acts and feels like when it is well. For example: Does your group have a lot of trust between members? Is there a lot of activity and energy? Are people all participating in some way? Is there a healthy level of respectful difference? Are we making progress toward our vision?

What does your program look, act and feel like when it is "well?"

_____

_____

_____

_____

Group On-Going Maintenance List

There are many factors that contribute to maintaining wellness in the group. This list could include things like weekly or daily check-ins, regular meetings, keeping the meeting space organized, being prepared, responding to calls and E-mails, or things like patience, being non-judgmental and a willingness to work through conflict.

What does your program or group need to do on an on-going basis to maintain "wellness" in your organization?

_____

_____

_____

_____

Triggers

The next section is triggers. Triggers for programs or groups are unexpected things that happen that are upsetting in some way. Group triggers might include discrimination against the group or people in the group, people being rude to each other, funding difficulties, loss of space, someone in the group having a difficult time, and power struggles. When the program is triggered, people may find that there is more gossip, more "posseing" (cliques of people ganging up on each other), and more assumptions. In a worst case scenario, triggers could lead to re-enactment dynamics (Chapter 7) where people tend to fall into roles with each other based on a set of inaccurate assumptions that are guided by people's personal histories. It is particularly important to recognize these dynamics as soon as they start to occur.

List some possible triggers that might upset your group or program:

_____

_____

_____

_____

The next step is to take action to prevent group "meltdown". Some of the things programs have done are:

- Call a membership meeting
- Do a "power analysis" in which people role play the dynamics of the program and then analyze "where the power is now".
- Review the values of the program
- Create a safe forum where people can acknowledge how they might be contributing to the problem
- Work together to find a solution
- Expression of feelings and emotions
- Non-judgmental support

What will your group/program need to do to get itself back on its feet if it is triggered?

_____

_____

Early Warning Signs

Early warning signs are subtle signs that things are not going well—the kinds of things we often overlook. However, if we pay attention to these signs and take action when they come up, we can often prevent further difficulties. These early warning signs may be the result of triggers. Or it may be hard to tell why they are happening. The reason may not be as important as realizing that things are not going well and taking corrective action. Some signs that things are not going well include gossiping, nitpicking, formation of cliques, people being rude to each other, impatience, and poor attendance.

What would be some early warning signs that your group is beginning to have difficulty?

When members of the group notice these early warning signs, taking action will help the group return to 'what it is like when it is well" and working toward its vision. Refer to your list of Wellness Tools for ideas. Some options might include: holding a special meeting to discuss the situation, mutual sharing, problem solving, having a retreat or doing a fun group activity.

List the actions your group could take if it noticed early warning signs.

When Things are Breaking Down

When things are breaking down is that time when things have gotten much worse. It may even feel like things are really starting to fall apart. Some signs that things are breaking down include: staff turnover, membership dropping, conflict that is not being addressed, blaming, people threatening each other with complaints or grievances, extreme "power trips" and members treating each other badly.

What is happening in your program when things are breaking down?

Sometimes groups try to fix things at this stage by creating more rules, posting lots of signs, and establishing stronger hierarchy in an attempt to "get things under control." Unfortunately these strategies will only serve to alienate people and/or maintain an unhealthy power dynamic.

At this time programs must really do some deep critical reflection. It is rarely only one thing that is contributing to this dynamic and it will take patience, humility, and integrity to get things back on track. Sometimes programs will close regular operations for a couple of days and instead invite all members to review program goals and values. At other times, groups may celebrate or have a party in the hopes of bringing people back together to remember all the good that they've accomplished. Still others may work with a mediator to try to get all "stories" out on the table.

What will your program need to do to get back on its feet when things breaking down?

_____

_____

_____

_____

Crisis

It is always our hope that we will figure out what to do before reaching a crisis. However, and unfortunately, crises happen entirely too often in our peer programs. This may be because peer programs are often under funded, understaffed, and working uphill against the dominant system. Indicators that the group is in a crisis include people suddenly quitting, threatening lawsuits, seemingly irresolvable conflict, and individuals or the board taking control away from the group.

What would be the signs that your group is in crisis? Perhaps your group has been in crisis before. What was that like?

_____

_____

_____

_____

At this time it is absolutely crucial that all key people in the organization revisit the mission and vision of the program. A facilitated evaluation group where everyone gets a chance to speak is important. Power dynamics must be analyzed and all key people must be willing to give and receive critical feedback. Perhaps people can make specific commitments about things they are willing to try. Looking back at how the group has survived crisis in the past may help you in thinking about what to do in another crisis situation.

What will your organization do to move through crisis?

_____

_____

_____

_____

When the organization or group has worked through these steps, they may want to have a meeting or several meetings to decide if they like their WRAP or if they want to change it in some way.

In order for WRAP to be effective, it needs to be reviewed regularly. The group could decide to review their WRAP weekly or monthly as part of an on-going assessment process and to keep the group moving forward. If action is needed the group can decide how that will happen. Before long, members of the group will become very familiar with the plan and will know what to do to keep the group well, will notice triggers and signs that things are not going well, and take action to improve the situation. Often the process of developing the WRAP is consciousness raising for the group and the group generally tends to "work better" and move more easily and quickly toward its vision.

Chapter 20
Final Thoughts

We hope this book has introduced you to many new thoughts, ideas, concepts and strategies for using WRAP and peer support together, and for any other mental health related work you are doing either personally or as part of an organization. Perhaps it went further than that, helping you and others begin to create positive changes in your lives and community.

Creating lasting change and doing things in new and different ways takes time. It is not possible to do it all at once. Change is often accompanied by feelings of discomfort, anxiety and fear. It often feels easier to do things the way we have been doing them, even if that doesn't feel right or is not very helpful. Try not to get discouraged. Begin with what feels most important to all of you at the time. Perhaps it is critical that you move from a "mental patient culture" to a wellness and recovery culture. Perhaps it is relinquishing control over some aspect of a program or project. Maybe it's getting together and really practicing shared decision-making. It may even be as simple as listening more closely to what others are saying.

If we take the risk and make room for carefully considered change, the rewards can be great. We can ease this process by understanding, supporting, and being honest with each other, even when we are upset. In addition, on-going discussion and refinement of proposed changes will ease the process and assure that things are done in ways that truly represent peer support and WRAP values and ethics.

The on-going assessment of yourself, your group or your organization is essential. If you are doing this work yourself, keep a journal of your progress. Use it as a tool to help you reflect on what you are doing and to decide what else you want to do and how you want to do it. If you are working with a group, organization or program, schedule regular meetings to assess what has been done and to make plans for the future. Keep careful records of your progress for easy reference when making decisions.

This book is not the final word. But we believe it is a step in the right direction. As you begin using the information and ideas in this manual, you will discover that there are even better ways of doing things. That's great! An on-going process of action and evaluation will support all changes. Everyone will benefit.

And last, it feels important to re-emphasize the value of building supportive relationships. Many of us who have had mental health related difficulties have a hard time building and keeping relationships, or even having enough trust to begin a relationship. It is very hard work. And yet it is crucial. Using WRAP and peer support and the values and ethics that guide them, we can overcome many of the barriers that have kept us trapped in roles that perpetuate the mental illness culture. We can move forward together and create the lives we want for ourselves. Quite honestly, we can change the world!

Appendices

Appendix A
Defining Peer Support

Shery Mead
March 2003

Peer support is a system of giving and receiving help founded on key principles of respect, shared responsibility, and mutual agreement of what is helpful. Peer support is not based on psychiatric models and diagnostic criteria. It is about understanding another's situation empathically through the shared experience of emotional and psychological pain. When people find affiliation with others whom they feel are "like" them, they feel a connection. This connection, or affiliation, is a deep, holistic understanding based on mutual experience where people are able to "be" with each other without the constraints of traditional (expert/patient) relationships. Further, as trust in the relationship builds, both people are able to respectfully challenge each other when they find themselves re-enacting old roles. This allows members of the peer community to try out new behaviors with one another and move beyond previously held self-concepts built on disability, diagnosis, and trauma worldview. The Stone Center refers to this as "mutual empowerment" (Stiver & Miller, 1998).

Peer support starts with the basic assumption that meaning and perception are created within the context of culture and relationships. Our self-definition, how we understand and interpret our experiences and how we relate to others is created and developed from the direct and indirect messages we get from others and the messages we get from dominant cultural beliefs and assumptions. We find that many of us who have used mental health services have been told what we "have," how "it" will be treated and how we must think about arranging our lives around this "thing." We have then begun to see our lives as a series of problems or "symptoms" and we have forgotten that there might be other ways to interpret our experiences. Because of this we have felt different and alone and "other-than" much of our lives, leaving us in relationships that have been less than mutually empowering and more often than not, destructive and infantilizing. We have learned to understand our experiences as signs of illness while burying histories of past violence and abuse. We have lost our power and our choices in most relationships. We have learned to either 'act as if,' or we have become dependent on professional interpretation of our every day experiences. It is not uncommon for us to then offer (and ask for) help based on this model.

Peer support training can help develop our ability to think critically about "who we've become." Training helps us learn to sit with discomfort while we explore the relational dynamics that have kept us stuck, and also helps us look at our own reactivity. It is helpful to understand people's "hot spots," and the kinds of situations that feel comfortable, tolerable, or absolutely intolerable so they can learn to negotiate power rather than take it. This then allows us to normalize what has been named as abnormal because of other people's discomfort (Dass & Gorman, 1985). Discovering this in a peer community reveals a different way of understanding our behaviors and presents an excellent framework to explore personal and relational change

One of the more significant (and dramatic) practices has been the development of peer run crisis respite programs. Theses programs emerged as an alternative to traditional psychiatric hospitalization (Mead & Hilton, 2002) and have been at the cutting edge of developing new practices for responding to crisis. They are essentially grounded in the knowledge that crisis can be transforming, that mutually supportive relationships provide necessary connection, and that new contexts offer new ways of thinking about one's experience. Rather than objectifying and naming the crisis experience in relation to the construct of illness (e.g. "You're getting sick again") people pro-actively and dialogically create a plan that serves as a guideline, and reminder, as to what kinds of interactions and activities will support a positive outcome for everyone. Out of this shared dynamic a sense of trust is built and the crisis can emerge as an opportunity to create new meaning around the experience while offering people mutually respectful relationships. As trust builds in the relationships and people feel valued, new ways of thinking, doing, and living become possible. The situation is shared rather than "handled," and it offers an opportunity for tremendous community growth.

Peer support programs must also challenge the current system's approach to how people with histories of abuse are treated. The devastating impact of abuse must be recognized for what it is and not viewed as psychiatric pathology or biological brain disorders. Through peer support services we can offer each other relationships that are respectful of our experiences, our ways of communicating, and how we have learned to tell our story. We can challenge each other to both face and to move beyond these stories and patterns. We can build new community norms that replace the illness environments that have kept us trapped. Finally, we can conscientiously name and expose the cultural violence that caused us to end up in these institutions. If we can learn to tell our stories in new ways, we can create communities where the sanctioned outcomes include non-compliance to "mental patient" identities or expectations, rejection of unhelpful treatment regimens, the questioning of overuse of medication, and speaking out about the prevalence of trauma and abuse. Finally, we can to call into question whose "problem" it really is.

It is no small feat for peer programs to develop this level of critical self-awareness. We are asking people to act in ways that are not instinctual and we are operating on a level of discomfort that shakes our very realities. It is here however, in community, that narrative becomes transformed. This means an entirely new interpretive framework for our construction of crisis/problem and our construction of help. In other words, we begin to understand change and learning not as an individual process, but rather one where we continuously construct knowledge from actions and reactions, conversations and the on-going building of consensus. Rather than thinking about personal symptom reduction we are talking about real social change.

Appendix B
Trauma and Peer Support:
Healing and Social Action

Shery Mead
May 2002

Those of us with histories of past trauma often feel "other-than." We have been told again and again that something is wrong with us, that we're "crazy," that it was our fault, and that we're bad. We have learned that our very lives are dependent on NOT trusting ourselves. We learn that what we know – based on what we see, feel and experience is not "true." What has become our truth – what is our reality – has been defined or "named" by others – not by us. Our instinctive feelings of terror, anger, and despair have never been accepted or acceptable and so our feelings and perceptions become linked to the "truth" that we have embodied. It is with these beliefs that we have sought mental health treatment for "our problems." If we have been lucky (and economically privileged) we may have found treatment that supports us in finding and rebuilding our voice, and helps us to move away from seeing ourselves as "the problem". If we've not been so lucky, our actions (or others' assessment of our actions) may have lead us to further abuse in terms of forced treatment, locked doors, physical restraints, and debilitating medications. Either way, we have been labeled with a psychiatric diagnosis and our experience has become further embedded in the "self as problem," and our pain as a symptom to be treated. We again have learned to view ourselves and our experiences through others' eyes, and we learn to believe that we are "mentally ill". Peer support can offer a fundamentally different framework for understanding our experiences and perceptions of our past, present, and future. It can provide us with opportunities to find new ways of understanding our world and our experiences and of finding new ways to respond to it. In peer support we can learn to form relationships outside of the definition or context of "illness" and to talk about the effects of trauma and abuse in our lives. We can share our stories with each other and we can begin to question how and why other people have learned to tell their stories in the ways that they do. We can begin to listen to each other in new ways, hearing the story rather than evaluating and assessing the problem. We can be witnesses to each other's pain. And most importantly we can validate the reality of each other's feelings, perceptions, and experiences. These conversations can influence the ways in which we respond to the situations we face, the ways we think about things, and can ultimately lead to our healing. As we challenge the naming of our experience by others we shake the whole foundation of a trauma worldview, and we begin to identify the larger cultural context in which we have been situated. As we unite in shared experiences and begin to expose the very structures that have kept us silenced, we find that "doing" social action becomes inextricably linked to healing — personally, socially and culturally. It is through this collective healing that real change happens, healing in fact that may prevent the "creation" of future mental patients.

Appendix C
Crisis as an Opportunity for Growth and Change

Shery Mead
September 2001

The concept of crisis in mental health is an interesting one. In spite of the fact that many traditional theorists have viewed crisis as an opportunity for growth and as an essential experience in the context of one's development (Erikson, 1976), we in mental health want to medicate it, lock it up, and restrain it. We have forgotten that perhaps there is something we can learn from this experience, something that will enable us to "do" it differently and understand ourselves in new ways.

Many of us at times have felt out of control, that our pain was more than we could manage, and even that life was not worth living. It has left us feeling isolated, alone, different and "crazy." It is not something that most of us want to go through again and again. And yet, we have been told and have come to believe that it is something that "happens" to us because of our illness. We are told that we are "decompensating" and that the goal is to return to a "pre-morbid" state. And so we go through life afraid of when "it" will happen next, believing that we must be careful not to get "stressed." Believing that we are fragile and out of control without our medications and our services. Instead of living life, we learn to avoid it as if it were dangerous. We have come to believe this because our experiences have been named for us. We are no longer individuals with unique perspectives but rather a set of generic symptoms that need a generic treatment. Though being labeled has been helpful to some, others of us have found it debilitating and limiting.

Peer support can offer a fundamentally different approach to crisis in that there are fewer assumptions about what it is people are experiencing. People may compare stories and strategies and ways of making meaning, but in the end, no one person has the power to name or to treat. Following is a way of thinking about being with people, even through very difficult times, that honors crisis as an opportunity to learn and grow and, most importantly, stay connected.

1. **Building mutual relationships.** It is only in relationships that are constantly negotiated that we build mutual respect and trust. When we consider that both of us have needs and expertise, we learn from each other while taking chances in becoming more vulnerable and consequently more "whole." As we take new risks in relationship, we find ourselves breaking out of old roles and assumptions, opening doors to self and relational discoveries that we never before knew existed.

2. **Being with "big" feelings."** We are not a culture that has a lot of tolerance for intensity or "big feelings." We tend to want to calm people down or make it stop

because *we* are uncomfortable. In peer support we can recognize that people have a lot of big feelings and they aren't all dangerous, they are in fact, rich with information.

3. **Understanding the "story."** I've always thought it was interesting that when people were having tough times, they were always asked what was wrong with them. What if, for example, we asked, "What happened to you?" Could we begin to understand the ways in which people's versions of their own stories impact the way they make meaning of their experiences now?

4. **Sharing ways that "stories" are understood.** One of the most valuable aspects of peer support is our ability to share our stories with each other. It's amazing to me what happens the first time we realize that we're not the only person who's been through some of these things. We can hear how each of us has learned to think about ourselves and can share strategies that take our <u>whole</u> story into account.

5. **Challenging the current story.** When trusting relationships develop and when both people are in control of the relationship, we can gently begin to challenge the ways each of us have learned to make meaning of our experiences. We can let each other know what works for us and what doesn't. Perhaps we are not decompensating—maybe we're justifiably angry and we don't know ways to express it. Perhaps we're not in suicidal depression; maybe we just feel tremendous shame and guilt for things we learned to believe were "our fault." When people compare and share, inevitably new stories are created and relationships deepen.

6. **Creating a new, shared story.** As relationships deepen we tend to take more risks, share our vulnerabilities and try on ways of "seeing" that were not previously available to us. We find ourselves in the process of examining our own beliefs and assumptions and we continuously try these out in relationship. We find that we are growing through the context of relationship. There are no limits to the possibilities because there are no static roles. We have the opportunity to be vulnerable and strong, helper and helped. We find that others are finding hope through our successes and that they are taking new risks.

Peer support is a culture of healing. As people practice new ways of "being" through even the most difficult times, possibilities for breaking old patterns and creating new opportunities are endless. Crisis then becomes just another word for re-defining our experience and ourselves, and instead of needing to be locked up, we can begin to break free.

Appendix D
Rights, Research & Liberation

Shery Mead
July 18, 2001

By and large, mental health research has been designed, conducted and analyzed by professional researchers working for academic institutions. Methods are generally quantitative and based on the measurement of pre-conceived constructs (e.g. reduced symptom severity, relapses and re-hospitalizations, improved social and vocational functioning etc.). Little is done to increase our understanding about the importance of culture, meaning, context, politics, and power, and few studies are conducted (let alone, read) by people who are directly affected by the research outcomes.

Most qualitative research methods focus on the meaning people make of their particular experiences and the ways in which meaning is negotiated through various relationships. Particular attention is paid to the cultures within which people live and the context within which experiences occur (historical, social, etc). Particular attention is also given to positions of power and privilege, language, and the dominant assumptions that contribute to the ways in which people describe their experiences. Often, people who are the "subjects" of the research are also the primary or co-researchers, and instead of professing value neutrality and objectivity, are explicit about creating change and challenging assumptions.

At a time, in mental health, when we are talking about "paradigm shifts" we forget that our methods and practices of research must also shift. Instead of focusing on individual illness constructs, we must focus on relationships, meaning, and social change (Mead & Hilton, 2001). Story telling is one way to broaden our discussion and our insights.

Storytelling has long been recognized as a way of describing one's self, differentiating one's self from other people, and a way of making connections with others. The way stories are told is influenced by who is listening, the questions that are being asked, when and where the story is being told and how the storyteller hopes to impact the listener. Stories that are told in groups are impacted by each other and can help elicit some of the "yet to be told" stories. In other words, stories are a relational, dynamic phenomenon that can allow people to challenge their self-images and contribute to the ways in which their listeners/ researchers/readers must challenge their own stories and the cultures within which their stories are constructed (Mead & Hilton, 2001). Following is example of this process.

A meeting was held at a Peer Support center to develop "outcome measures" for the peer center. I was invited to facilitate the process and to explain action and narrative research. To help us get away from the traditional research roles, I asked the group to talk about their experiences with other research projects they'd been involved with. Responses were unilateral; people had been "subjects" of the research, saw themselves in illness roles, had rarely seen research reports (which were difficult to understand at best), and were quite sure that the outcomes of the research had made no difference in their lives. Furthermore, they had wanted to provide the "right" answers (even when the questions were nebulous), they had felt "less than," and had felt uncomfortable knowing nothing about the researchers background, or whether they could ask about it. Research itself was intimidating.

I asked if people wanted to define for themselves, what Peer Support meant and how it should be written about or evaluated. Although there was some confusion and discomfort about the process, the group signed on. It was not going to be easy, I pointed out, to be both experiencing the difference Peer Support makes in your life while reflecting on that experience and the experience of others. We started talking about some of the ways in which the peer center had already made a difference in people's lives.

This group had recently written, produced and participated in a play about stigma. Though the content of the play was important, some of the other outcomes were surprising and life changing. People told stories about getting "symptomatic" before a production and wanting to quit. As they talked among each other and with other members of the center, they began to realize, that in a different language, it might have been their version of stage fright. In fact this experience was the topic of the play and they were living it. By going through with the performance, not only did they push past their perceived limitations but they were also able to challenge their understandings and meanings of their "symptoms." At the same time they put forth a living narrative, which challenged the audience's assumptions and understandings. As the play continued to be performed, it was less scripted and more evolving. Participants began to realize that the play was less about stigma education and more about role changes, relational growth and social change. By telling their stories in new ways again and again, stories became re-constructions and the peer center began to make some cultural shifts and build a new community identity.

After sharing the story about their play we talked about some of the ways people had chosen to tell their story in the play and how they thought they had learned to tell that story. We talked about how their self-perception, relationships and understanding of "mental illness" had changed and we talked about how we wanted to document and analyze this "data." Emerging themes we chose to focus on included changes in language, risk taking, building deeper relationships, challenging some of the traditional mental health practices, and becoming more involved in the peer center as well as the larger community. The process of exploration needed to include taking weekly actions (risks in relationships, trying new things, challenging aspects of their treatment etc.) and reflecting upon why they had chosen those particular actions, as well as the changes those actions evoked. The format would be journal, and/or taped discussions. "Validity" testing would be done by different members of the research group playing the role of devil's advocate (Reason, 1989). Through this process, other members would be part of the conversations, asked to join in the research, and a community "story" would be written. Our hope was that, because theatre worked so well for this community, other artistic forms might become part of the research.

This is only one example of the ways in which research can expose more complex systems at work. For mental health this has implications that have, up to this point, been seriously overlooked. Those of us who have been labeled with mental illness exist in cultures where meaning is imposed on us. We have taken on roles and identities that keep us separate and feeling "other-than." If our research is to have real meaning, we must all become "reflective practitioner" researchers (Schon, 1983) on ourselves and with each other. We must not let ourselves be reduced to arbitrary constructions and we must not let someone else tell our stories and have control over who we become. The goal of our research must be to empower all those involved (researchers, participants, and readers) to move away from the "reified" conclusions that traditional research has drawn (Bentz and Shapiro, 1998). In that, we must all be willing to challenge our assumptions and perceptions, have new "conversations," and continuously build new ways of creating knowledge together.

Appendix E
Crisis Plan

Part 1 What I'm like when I'm feeling well

Describe yourself when you are feeling well.

_____

_____

_____

_____

_____

_____

_____

_____

_____

_____

_____

Part 2 Symptoms

Describe those symptoms that would indicate to others that they need to take over full responsibility for your care and make decisions in your behalf.

_____

_____

_____

_____

_____

_____

_____

_____

_____

_____

_____

_____

Part 3 Supporters

List those people you want to take over for you when the symptoms you listed above are obvious. They can be family members, friends or health care professionals. Have at least five people on your list of supporters. You may want to name some people for certain tasks like taking care of the children or paying the bills and others for tasks like staying with you and taking you to health care appointments.

Name	Connection/role	Phone number

There may be health care professionals or family members that have made decisions that were not according to your wishes in the past. They could inadvertently get involved if you don't include the following:

I do not want the following people involved in any way in my care or treatment:

Name	Why you do not want them involved (optional)

Settling Disputes Between Supporters

You might like to include a section that describes how you want possible disputes between supporters settled. For instance, you may want to say that a majority need to agree, or that a particular person or two people make the determination.

Part 4 Medication

Physician _____ Phone Number _____

Physician #2 _____ Phone Number _____

Pharmacy _____ Phone Number _____

List the medications you are currently using and why you are taking them.

_____

_____

_____

_____

List those medications you would prefer to take if medications or additional medications became necessary and why you would choose those.

_____

_____

_____

_____

List those medications that would be acceptable to you if medications became necessary and why you would choose those.

_____

_____

_____

_____

List those medications that should be avoided and give the reasons.

_____

_____

_____

_____

Part 5 Treatments

List treatments that help reduce your symptoms and when they should be used.

_____

_____

_____

_____

_____

List treatments you would want to avoid.

_____

_____

_____

_____

Part 6 Home/Community Care/Respite Center

Set up a plan so that you can stay at home or in the community and still get the care you need.

_____

_____

_____

_____

_____

Part 7 Treatment Facilities

List treatment facilities where you prefer to be treated or hospitalized if that becomes necessary.

_____

_____

_____

_____

List treatment facilities you want to avoid.

_____

_____

_____

_____

_____

Part 8 Help from others

List those things that others can do for you that would help reduce your symptoms or make you more comfortable.

_____
_____
_____
_____
_____
_____

List those things you need others to do for you and who you want to do these things.

What I need done　　　　　　**Who I'd like to do it**

_____
_____
_____
_____
_____

List those things that others might do, or have done in the past, that would not help or might even worsen your symptoms.

_____
_____
_____
_____
_____

Part 9 Inactivating the Plan

Describe symptoms, lack of symptoms or actions that indicate supporters no longer need to use this plan.

_____
_____
_____
_____
_____

You can help assure that your crisis plan will be followed by signing it in the presence of two witnesses. It will further increase its potential for use if you appoint and name a durable power of attorney.

I developed this plan on (date) _____

with the help of _____

Any plan with a more recent date supersedes this one.

Signed _____ Date _____

Witness _____ Date _____

Witness _____ Date _____

Attorney _____ Date _____

Durable Power of Attorney (if you have one) _____

Phone Number _____

Appendix F
Post Crisis Plan

I will know that I am "out of the crisis" and ready to use this post crisis plan when I:

_____

_____

_____

_____

How I would like to feel when I have recovered from this crisis:
(You may want to refer to the first section of your Wellness Recovery Action Plan—What I am Like When I am Well. This may be different from what you feel like when you are well—your perspective may have changed in this crisis.)

_____

_____

_____

_____

Post Recovery Supporters List

I would like the following people to support me if possible during this post crisis time:

Who: Phone number: What I need them to do:

_____   _____   _____

_____   _____   _____

_____   _____   _____

_____   _____   _____

_____   _____   _____

If you are being discharged from a treatment facility, do you have a place to go that is safe and comfortable?   ___ yes ___ no

If not, what do you need to do to insure that you have a safe comfortable place to go?

_____

_____

Arriving at Home
(if you have been hospitalized or away from home)

If you have been hospitalized, your first few hours at home are very important. Will you feel safe and be safe at home? ___yes ___no

If your answer is no, what will you do to insure that you will feel and be safe at home?

_____

_____

_____

_____

_____

I would like _____ or _____
to take me home.

I would like _____ or _____
to stay with me.

When I get home I would like to _____ or

_____

If the following things were in place, it would ease my return:

_____

_____

_____

_____

Things I must take care of as soon as I get home:

_____

_____

_____

_____

Things I can ask someone else to do for me:

_____

_____

_____

_____

Things that can wait until I feel better:

_____
_____
_____
_____
_____

Things I need to do for myself every day while I am recovering from crisis:

_____
_____
_____
_____
_____

Things I might need to do every day while I am recovering from this crisis:

_____
_____
_____
_____
_____

Things and people I need to avoid while I am recovering from this crisis:

_____
_____
_____
_____
_____

Signs that I may be beginning to feel worse:
(anxiety, excessive worry, overeating, sleep disturbances)

_____
_____
_____
_____

Wellness tools I will use if I am starting to feel worse:
(star those that you must do, the others are choices)

_____
_____
_____
_____

What do I need to do to prevent further repercussions from this crisis—and when I will do these things:

_____

_____

_____

_____

_____

People I need to thank:

Person:	When I will thank them:	How I will thank them:
_____	_____	_____
_____	_____	_____
_____	_____	_____
_____	_____	_____
_____	_____	_____

People I need to apologize to:

Person:	When I will apologize:	How I will apologize:
_____	_____	_____
_____	_____	_____
_____	_____	_____
_____	_____	_____
_____	_____	_____

People with whom I need to make amends:

Person:	When I will make amends:	How I will make amends:
_____	_____	_____
_____	_____	_____
_____	_____	_____
_____	_____	_____
_____	_____	_____

Medical, legal, or financial issues that need to be resolved:

Issue: How I plan to resolve this issue:

_____   _____

_____   _____

_____   _____

_____   _____

_____   _____

Things I need to do to prevent further loss:
(canceling credit cards, getting official leave from work if it was abandoned, cutting ties with destructive friends, etc.)

_____

_____

_____

_____

Signs that this post crisis phase is over and I can return to using my Daily Maintenance Plan as my guide to things to do for myself every day:

_____

_____

_____

_____

Changes in the first 4 sections my Wellness Recovery Action Plan that might help prevent such a crisis in the future:

_____

_____

_____

_____

Changes in my crisis plan that might ease my recovery:

_____

_____

_____

_____

Changes I want to make in my lifestyle or life goals:

_____

_____

_____

_____

What did I learn from this crisis?

_____

_____

_____

_____

Are there changes I want or need to make in my life as a result of what I have learned?

_____

_____

_____

_____

If so, when and how will I make these changes?

_____

_____

_____

_____

Timetable for Resuming Responsibilities

Responsibility: _____

Who has been doing this while I was in crisis:_____

While I am resuming this responsibility, I need (who): _____

     to_____

Plan for resuming:

_____

_____

_____

_____

Responsibility: _____

Who has been doing this while I was in crisis:_____

While I am resuming this responsibility, I need (who): _____

    to_____

Plan for resuming:

_____

_____

_____

_____

Responsibility: _____

Who has been doing this while I was in crisis:_____

While I am resuming this responsibility, I need (who): _____

    to_____

Plan for resuming:

_____

_____

_____

_____

Responsibility: _____

Who has been doing this while I was in crisis:_____

While I am resuming this responsibility, I need (who): _____

    to_____

Plan for resuming:

_____

_____

_____

_____

Appendix G
References

Bentz, V., and Shapiro, J., (1998). *Mindful Inquiry in Social Research.* Sage Publications: Thousand Oaks, CA.

Bloom, S., (1997). *Creating sanctuary: Toward the Evolution of Sane Societies.* Routledge: NY.

Copeland, M. E. (2001). *The Depression Workbook: A Guide for Living with Depression and Manic Depression* (2nd ed.). Oakland, CA: New Harbinger Publications.

Copeland, M.E. & Harris, M. *Healing the Trauma of Abuse.* Oakland, CA: New Harbinger Publications.

Copeland, M. E. (1994). *Living Without Depression and Manic Depression.* Oakland, CA: New Harbinger Publications.

Copeland, M. E. (1999). *The Loneliness Workbook.* Oakland, CA: New Harbinger Publications.

Copeland, M. E. (1997, Revised 2001). *Wellness Recovery Action Plan.* Brattleboro, VT: Peach Press.

Copeland, M. E. (2000). *Winning Against Relapse.* Brattleboro, VT: Peach Press.

Herman, J.L. (1992). *Trauma and Recovery.* New York: Basic Books.

MacNeil, C. (2003). *A Community of Support.* Brunswick, ME: Sweetser.

Mead, S., Hilton, D., Curtis L. (2001). *Peer Support: A Theoretical Perspective.* Psychiatric Rehabilitation Journal, 5(2), 134 – 141

Mead, S., and Hilton, D., (unpublished paper 2001). *Peer Support: A Systemic Approach to Mental Health.*

Reason, P., (ed.) (1988). *Human Inquiry In Action: Developments In New Paradigm Research.* Sage Publications: Thousand Oaks, CA.

Schon, D.A., (1983). *The Reflective Practitioner.* Jossey-Bass: San Francisco.

Self-Help Resources by Mary Ellen Copeland, PhD

The Depression Workbook: A Guide to Living with Depression and
    Manic Depression Second Edition _____ copies at $19.95

Fibromyalgia and Chronic Myofascial Pain Syndrome: A Survival Manual with Devin Starlanyl _____ copies at $19.95

Healing the Trauma of Abuse: A Women's Workbook with Maxine Harris, PhD _____ copies at $24.95

Living Without Depression and Manic Depression: A Guide to Maintaining Mood Stability _____ copies at $21.95

The Loneliness Workbook _____ copies at $16.95

Recovering from Depression: A Workbook for Teens with Stuart Copans, MD _____ copies at $24.95

WRAP: Wellness Recovery Action Plan   1-9 copies, $10 each. _____ copies at $10.00

WRAP: Wellness Recovery Action Plan for People with Dual Diagnosis _____ copies at $10.00

WRAP-Spanish Version- Plan de Acción para la Recuperación del Bienestar _____ copies at $10.00
WRAP Quantity pricing: 10-99 copies, $8 each. 100+ copies, $7 each. Call for shipping quote.

WRAP Software Contains both adult and teen versions _____ copies at $19.95

WRAP and Peer Support Manual: Personal, Group & Program Development with Shery Mead _____ copies at $40.00

Winning Against Relapse: A Workbook of Action Plans for Recurring Health & Emotional Problems
    Expanded version of WRAP with suggestions for group work _____ copies at $16.95

The Worry Control Workbook _____ copies at $16.95

Facilitator Manual: Mental Health Recovery including WRAP _____ copies at $129.00
    with CD of transparencies and complete instructions for teaching WRAP ($8 shipping)

Advanced Mental Health Recovery Manual: Leading a WRAP Facilitator Training _____ copies at $60.00

Community Links: Pathways to Recovery Program Implementation Manual with CD _____ copies at $70.00

Video and Audio

Creating Wellness Workshop Video Series: produced by Mental Illness Education Project

❃ Key Concepts for Mental Health video _____ copies at $39.95

❃ Wellness Tools video _____ copies at $39.95

❃ Developing a Wellness Recovery Action Plan (WRAP) video _____ copies at $39.95

Wellness Tools audio CD _____ copies at $19.95

WRAP: Step-by-Step audio CD _____ copies at $19.95

Total number of items _____ **Subtotal $**_____

Shipping/Handling: $4 for the first item + $1 for each additional item _____

Total amount due (for resource items and shipping costs)_____

Name _____Organization _____

Address_____

City and State _____ Zip _____

Phone_____ E-mail _____

Make checks payable to Mary Ellen Copeland.

( ) MasterCard ( ) Visa Card # _____ Expires _____

Mail order to: Mary Ellen Copeland, PO Box 301, West Dummerston, VT 05357-0301 USA

mentalhealthrecovery.com Phone 802-425-3660 FAX 802-425-5580 books@mentalhealthrecovery.com

MENTAL HEALTH RECOVERY
Curriculum
including

Wellness Recovery Action Planning

Facilitator
Training Manual

By Mary Ellen Copeland, PhD

The *Facilitator Training Manual* with CD-ROM is an invaluable resource for anyone who is committed to sharing mental health self-help recovery information.

This comprehensive curriculum package includes:
- **Section I, Curriculum**: specific instructions for teaching recovery and WRAP in different circumstances and settings.
- **Section II, Transparencies**: both thumbnail sketches and a CD-Rom of over 200 workshop presentation transparencies.
- **Section III, Activities, Handouts and Discussion Topics**: suggestions for each topic, following the sequence of the transparencies, and handouts that may be copied and distributed.
- **Section IV, Resources**: an extensive listing of mental health resources for the facilitator.

The curriculum was originally designed for participants in training seminars. It has been revised to provide guidance to a broader audience of people teaching recovery who adhere to the values and guidelines outlined in the curriculum.

Facilitator Manual: Mental Health Recovery including WRAP   _____ copies at $129.00

Subtotal $ _____

Shipping/Handling: total # curriculum x $8.00 per item   _____

Total amount due   _____

Name _____

Address_____

City and State _____ Zip _____

Phone_____ e-mail _____

Make checks payable to Mary Ellen Copeland.

( ) Mastercard ( ) Visa Card # _____ Expires _____

Mail order to: Mary Ellen Copeland, PO Box 301, West Dummerston, VT 05357-0301

Phone 802-254-2092   FAX 802-257-7499

E-mail: books@mentalhealthrecovery.com   Web site: www.mentalhealthrecovery.com

Order Form

Intentional Peer Support: An Alternative Approach
        Shery Mead, MSW.......................... $30 US
        ($25 for 6 or more copies)

WRAP and Peer Support
        Mary Ellen Copeland and Shery Mead... $40 US
        ($35 for 6 or more copies)

Shipping and Handling : $2.50/ book or manual

Order form

Name: _____

Address_____

         _____

         _____

Title	Number	Cost	S/H
_____	_____	_____	_____
_____	_____	_____	_____
_____	_____	_____	_____

TOTAL   _____

Credit Card Info

Type   _____   Name as it appears on card_____

Number _____

Exp date_____

Please contact Shery Mead at 603-469-3577 (phone and fax) or shery@mentalhealthpeers.com to order books. Remit payment to Shery Mead 302 Bean Rd Plainfield, NH 03781